William Henry Seward's
Quest to Save the Nation During the Secession Winter
(November 1860-April 1861)

William Henry Seward's
Quest to Save the Nation During the Secession Winter
(November 1860-April 1861)

C. Evan Stewart

Twelve Tables Press

ISBN: 978-1-946074-46-1

Twelve Tables Press
P.O. Box 568
Northport, New York 11768
www.twelvetablespress.com

10 9 8 7 6 5 4 3 2 1

Cover Art: Reprinted by Permission, Alamy.com 2026

To

John B. Barbour, Anne Fiske Barnes,
Mary Fiske Beck, Francis W. Coker Jr.
(my godparents)

and

Edwin W. Fiske Jr. and Jessie Boulton Fiske
(my third set of grandparents)

and

James H. McGlothlin and Patricia Dowd McGlothlin
(my parents-in-law)

Contents

Preface

Abraham Lincoln was the nation's greatest president. But that does not mean he was perfect. For example, his administration's record on curtailing civil liberties in the name of the war effort was pretty bad (see Chapters XVII and XVIII in *The Worst Supreme Court Decisions, Ever! (And Related Tales)* (Twelve Table Press 2024)).

After being elected president in November 1860 (with less than 40 percent of the popular vote), Lincoln faced a nation in existential crisis: South Carolina quickly seceded, with the other Deep South States following in short order. The fate of the Upper South States was precarious (at best), and the president-elect stayed in relative seclusion at his home in Illinois, waiting out the four months until he would be inaugurated on March 4, 1861.

What equipped Lincoln to deal with this crisis? He had been a trial lawyer and a local politician most of his life. He had spent an uneventful term in Congress more than a decade before, and had unsuccessfully run for the U.S. Senate twice. He had no executive experience of any kind. And besides those he had served with in Congress, he knew virtually none of the key players in Washington D.C., nor virtually any of the anti-secessionist leaders in the Upper South States.[1] As for those Lincoln chose for his Cabinet, it was a highly dysfunctional group of men—some of whom thought they should have been president instead, and all fiercely jealous of the others and their influence over the new and inexperienced president.[2] Not a pretty picture for a man trying to hold a country together and avoid a civil war.

In the winter of 1860-61, one man, William Henry Seward, Republican Senator from New York (the presumptive favorite for the 1860 Republican nomination for president; defeated by Lincoln on the third ballot), labored mightily to effectuate his plan to save the Union. Because of history's (and historians') heavy bias to portray Lincoln as almost a saint (see, for example, Jon Meacham's *And There Was Light: Abraham Lincoln and the American Struggle* (Random House 2022)), Seward's prodigious efforts have either been ignored, given short shrift, or looked upon as something less than honorable.[3]

This short book—based on original archival research and a comprehensive review of secondary sources—tells the story of Seward's efforts. Counterfactual history is always an iffy business. But Seward's "plan" did help to keep the Upper South States in the Union during the months before the president-elect became the president. And had his counsel been followed after March 4, perhaps the course of American history would have played out very differently.

This book will attempt to provide a complete explication of Seward's plan and his prodigious efforts to save the Union during the Secession Winter of November 1860 through April 1861.

Notes

1. As historian David Potter observed, in 1860 Lincoln was "a man of great undeveloped capacities and narrowly limited background. He was far more fit to become than to be President." *Lincoln and His Party in the Secession Crisis,* p. x (Louisiana State University Press 1995 (originally Yale University Press 1942)). And as Lincoln's greatest biographer, David Donald, wrote about his subject as the Secession Winter began: "All eyes now turned to Springfield, where an inexperienced leader with a limited acquaintance among members of his own party groped his way, on the basis of inadequate information, to formulate a policy for his new administration." *Lincoln,* p. 257 (Simon & Schuster 1996).

2. This dysfunctional group is well depicted in Doris Kearns Goodwin's *Team of Rivals: The Political Genius of Abraham Lincoln* (Simon & Schuster 2006); see also C. Evan Stewart, *The Worst Supreme Court Decisions, Ever! (And Related Tales)* (Chapter XXI) (Twelve Tables Press 2024). For those readers wanting a detailed look into this dysfunctional group, see *The Civil War Diary of Gideon Welles* (William Gienapp & Erica Gienapp eds.) (University of Illinois Press 2014).

3. The conventional/consensus history of the Secession Winter and Lincoln's primary/crucial role therein is represented by David Potter's classic book *Lincoln and His Party in the Secession Crisis* (cited above) (Seward's role during this period was that of Lincoln's "agent" in Washington); a more current (but consistent) approach is set forth in Harold Holzer's *Lincoln President-Elect: Abraham Lincoln and the Great Secession Winter 1860-1861* (Simon & Schuster 2008). Michael Burlingame's magisterial two volume *Abraham Lincoln: A Life* (Johns Hopkins University Press 2009) portrays Seward's efforts in a negative light (calling them "appeasement" and "one of the great mysteries of the secession crisis"); Kenneth Stampp was equally critical of Seward's efforts, see *And the War Came: The North and Secession Crisis, 1860-61*, p. 272 (Louisiana State University Press 1950) (Seward's efforts showed "incredible blindness"); as was Allan Nevins, see *The War for Union*, Vol. I, pp. 39, 27, 74 (Charles Scribner's Sons 1959-71) (Seward's policies of "appeasement" and peace "at any price" were evidence of "a profound moral defect"); (Potter deemed Seward "an enigma," who "followed a course which perplexed his contemporaries and has baffled historians"—pp. 182, 303). Most recently, British historian Nigel Hamilton has call Seward "an obviously treacherous individual ... [who engaged in] treason," and "a rank traitor"; not stopping there, Hamilton also labeled Seward

"not as Iago, but as Judas." *Lincoln vs. Davis: The War of the Presidents,* pp. 107, 123-25, 582-83 (Little, Brown and Company 2024).

Over 40 years ago, one prominent historian did weigh in on the other side of the debate, arguing that Seward's efforts "offered at a critical turning point in American history, merit[ed] a fresh assessment." See Daniel Crofts, "Secession Winter: William Henry Seward and the Decision for War," *New York History* (July 1984); see also Daniel Crofts, "The Union Party of 1861 and the Secession Crisis," *Perspectives in American History* (1977-78); Daniel Crofts, *Reluctant Confederates: Upper South Unionists in the Secession Crisis* (University of North Carolina Press 1987); Daniel Crofts's Introduction to Potter's book ("The riveting struggle over southern policy between Lincoln and Seward during the secession winter was one of the most dramatic confrontations in American history."—pp. xxv-xxvi); Daniel Crofts, "The Diary of a Public Man," *Civil War History* (2009). See also Patrick Sowle, "The Conciliatory Republicans During the Winter of Secession," pp. 511-12 (Ph.D. Dissertation) (Duke University 1963) (Potter misinterpreted the secession winter—to Potter it was "not as a period of bitter feuding between two Republican factions, but as a time in which Lincoln rallied the party behind his ideas about the crisis.... Seward is considered not Lincoln's rival, but his Washington agent."); Russell McClintock, *Lincoln and the Decision for War: The Northern Response to Secession* (University of North Carolina Press 2008); Lawrence Denton, *William Henry Seward and the Secession Crisis* (McFarland & Company 2009).

William Henry Seward's
Quest to Save the Nation During the Secession Winter
(November 1860-April 1861)

Chapter I

Leader of the Republican Party

William Henry Seward (1801-72) of Auburn, New York, was one of the most consequential Americans of the nineteenth century. Not only did he construct the blueprint for America's overseas expansion (e.g., acquiring the Guano Islands and Midway, brokering the greatest real estate deal in American history—"Seward's Folly," the purchase of Alaska from Russia in 1867 for $7.2 million, etc.), he was also a two-term governor of New York (1839-43), a U.S. senator (1849-61), and U.S. Secretary of State, an office he held through both the Lincoln and Johnson administrations (1861-69).[1]

Seward, in 1860, was also the acknowledged leader of the Republican Party and the clear front-runner for the party's presidential nomination that year. Seward could have had the nomination in 1856 (when the

Republican Party was still in formation as a potent political threat to the Democratic Party—in the Northern states), but he (and his political ally, mentor, and New York's political boss, Thurlow Weed (nicknamed "the Dictator")) thought 1856 would not be a winning year and they decided to wait four years.[2] Seward was so sure of his chances in 1860 that he spent more than half of 1859 (May to the end of December) touring Europe, where he was regularly welcomed as the soon-to-be president.[3]

The political environment in America to which Seward returned was not a happy one, principally because of John Brown's aborted attempt in 1859 to foment a slave insurrection by taking over the federal armory at Harpers Ferry, Virginia, as well as the political reality now dawning on Southern Fire-Eaters—that the Republican Party (with no Southern support) had a significant chance of winning the presidency in November of 1860. Many Southern politicians, because of Seward's prominent status (as well as his 1858 speech citing an "irrepressible conflict" between the free labor states and the slaveholding states),[4] took aim directly at the front-runner. Congressman Reuben Davis of Mississippi was a prime example:

> Gentlemen of the Republican Party, I warn you. Present your sectional candidate in 1860, elect him as the representative of your system of labor, take possession of the Government as your instrument in this "irrepressible conflict," and we of the South will tear the Constitution to pieces, and look to our guns for justice.[5]

Not only hoping to tamp down at least some of this hostility (and project a more moderate image)[6] but also to help the passage of a bill he introduced (on February 21, 1860, for the admission of Kansas as a state), Seward rose in the Senate on February 29 to give a widely anticipated speech to a packed Senate and overflowing galleries. Seward argued that his party posed no threat to the status of slavery in the Southern states and denounced John Brown's raid (adding that his execution was "necessary and just"). Seward then turned to the Southern threat(s) of secession:

> Those who seek to awaken the terrors of disunion … have too hastily considered the conditions under which they are to make their attempt. Who believes that a Republican administration and Congress could practice

> tyranny under a Constitution which interposes so many checks as ours?

And anticipating some editorial suggestions he would make a year later to Lincoln's Inaugural Address, Seward also spoke of the "bonds" that held the Union together and made it "inseparable and indivisible" (the "millions of fibers of millions of contented happy human hearts, binding by their affections, their ambitions and their best hopes").[7]

Seward's speech was widely praised in the Northern press as moderating his 1858 "irrepressible conflict" challenge to the South, but was not so perceived by the Southern press.[8] More problematic for an easy road to the nomination was the widespread (and highly praised) press that Lincoln was receiving for his February 27 speech at Cooper Union in New York City—a speech that Lincoln later said was critical to him becoming president.[9]

February of 1860 was an important month for an additional reason. On February 22, the Republican National Committee met in New York City to decide where to hold the national convention. Seward's people wanted New York; supporters of another leading contender, Ohio's Governor Salmon Chase, advocated for Ohio; and the third leading candidate's representative (on behalf of Edward Bates, former congressman from Missouri, who was backed by the politically powerful Blair family) wanted St. Louis. Norman Judd—the Illinois representative (and Lincoln's unannounced agent)—brokered a compromise: a city in a state not tied to any *leading* candidate should be the site; and so the Committee—just days before Lincoln's Cooper Union speech—agreed upon Chicago.[10] That decision would prove to be a significant nail in the coffin of Seward's (and Weed's) presidential plans.

Notes

1. The definitive biographies of Seward are Glyndon Van Deusen's 1967 book *William Henry Seward* (Oxford University Press) and Walter Stahr's *Seward: Lincoln's Indispensable Man* (Simon & Schuster 2012); see also Frederic Bancroft, *The Life of William H. Seward* (Harper & Row 1900); John M. Taylor, *William Henry Seward: Lincoln's Right Hand* (HarperCollins 1991), C. Evan Stewart, "Diplomat of the Civil War," *New York Archives* (Summer 2011); C. Evan Stewart, "William Henry Seward, 19th Century Advocate and Statesman," *Federal Bar Council News* (April 1998). For readers interested in understanding how Seward constructed the blueprint for America's overseas expansion, see Walter LaFeber's *The American Search for Opportunity, 1865-1913* (Cambridge University Press 1993) and Walter LaFeber's Presidential Address (to the Society for Historians of American Foreign Relations): "Technology and U.S.

Foreign Relations" in *Diplomatic History* (Winter 2000). See also Anders Stephanson, *Manifest Destiny: American Expansion and the Empire of Right*, pp. 58-63 (Hill and Wang 1995).

2. See Van Deusen, supra note 1, pp. 174-78; Stahr, supra note 1, pp. 159-60; Taylor, supra note 1, pp. 109-112. For definitive biographies of Weed, see Thurlow W. Barnes's *Memoir of Thurlow Weed* (Houghton Mifflin 1884) and Glydon Van Deusen's *Thurlow Weed: Wizard of the Lobby* (Little Brown and Company 1947).

As for Seward's front-running status, Frederic Bancroft expressed it as follows:

> The fact that Seward had been prominent so long, that for a decade he had no rival in the opinion of the progressive people of the North, that he had been in perfect harmony with the changing tendencies, first of the best Whigs and then of the best Republicans—these furnished opportunities for dangerous attacks upon him. Notwithstanding the numerous objections—some sincere by many specious—Seward was still the favorite of a very large majority of the Republican voters and politicians.

(supra note 1, p. 525).

Weed's commitment to Seward's political career is best exemplified by his May 15, 1858, letter to Seward, in which he wrote that making Seward president was "a purpose which for twenty years [has] engrossed my thoughts and controlled my action." Glyndon Van Deusen (ed.), "Thurlow Weed's Analysis of William Henry Seward's Defeat in the Republican Convention of 1860," *Mississippi Valley Historical Review*, p. 101 (1947). See also Daniel Crofts's

Reluctant Confederates: Upper South Unionists in the Secession Crisis, p. 217 (University of North Carolina Press 1987).

3. Seward's European travels in 1859 are best captured by his son's book, Frederick W. Seward, *Seward at Washington: 1846-61*, pp. 362-463 (Derby and Miller 1891) (which is the middle of a three-volume set of a memoir Seward's son authored). Stahr, by contrast, devotes three pages to Seward's trip (supra note 1, pp. 178-80). Before leaving for Europe, Seward traveled to Harrisburg, Pennsylvania, in April to meet with Republican Senator Simon Cameron, the leader of that state's party. Seward later reported to Weed that Cameron "told me all was right, He was for me, and Pennsylvania would be." Seward letter to Weed, April 11, 1859 (Weed Papers, University of Rochester). As we will see, Cameron's word was not his bond.

Franklin Roosevelt's Vice President, Henry Wallace, would also learn in 1944 that leaving the country for an extended period before a party's national convention can be a very expensive trip (to one's political career). See Ben Steil's *The World That Wasn't* (Avid Reader Press 2024).

4. For an explication of and context for Seward's famous "irrepressible conflict" speech, see Van Deusen, supra note 1, pp. 188-96, and Stahr, supra note 1, pp. 165-81; see also Robert Johannsen *Lincoln, The South, and Slavery*, pp. 69-99 (Louisiana State University Press 1991); Michael Holt, *The Election of 1860: A Campaign Fraught with Consequences*, pp. 22-23 (University Press of Kansas 2017). Seward had initially become famous nationally—and a targeted villain in the South—when he gave his first speech on the floor of the U.S. Senate on March 11, 1850. Opposing the Compromise of 1850 (Henry Clay's efforts to bring an end to conflict over the expansion of slavery), Seward countered the South's invoking the Constitution's

protections of slavery by citing to "A Higher Law." Van Deusen, supra note 1, pp. 113-28; Stahr, supra note 1, pp. 116-43. See also Michael Holt, *The Rise and Fall of the American Whig Party: Jacksonian Politics and the Onset of the Civil War*, pp. 489-93 (Oxford University Press 1999).

5. F. Seward, supra note 3, p. 442. For other Southern diatribes aimed at Seward, see id. pp. 444-46 (e.g., an advertisement in a Richmond Virginia newspaper offering $50,000 "for the head of William Henry Seward").

6. Notwithstanding the intensity of Southern rhetoric directed at Seward, in fact many Southern politicians were quite friendly and frequently socialized with him. Jefferson Davis, for example, was a good friend of Seward's. David Potter, *Lincoln and His Party in the Secession Crisis*, p. 25 (Louisiana State University Press 1995 (originally Yale University Press 1942)); Michael Holt, *The Election of 1860*, p. 90, supra note 4.

7. In fact, Seward argued (as he had earlier in a famous 1852 speech to the Senate) that the greater issue facing the country was finding a way(s) to bind the east and west coasts of America closer together through technology, trade, and immigration. See William H. Seward, *Commerce in the Pacific Ocean: Speech of William H. Seward, in the Senate of the United States, July 29, 1852* (Forgotten Books, Classic Reprint Series 2018); see also Van Deusen, supra note 1, pp. 147-49.

Jefferson Davis immediately rose in the Senate to respond to Seward: "But the Senator from New York invokes us by his love for the Union, and in the spirit of fraternity, I have nothing to object to the time in which he had addressed us, but I wish we could have acts instead of words.... If the Senator would show to us ... that we may rely on the pledge which he gives us that the Republican party ...

cannot trespass on the rights of any section, our faith might follow." *Jefferson Davis: The Essential Writings*, pp. 166-72 (William Cooper ed.) (Random House 2003).

8. F. Seward, supra note 3, pp. 443-46; Stahr, supra note 1, p. 184. The *New York Times* printed Seward's speech in its entirety in a special edition. The *New York Tribune* called it "[s]o calm in temper, so philosophic in statement, so comprehensive in grasp, so passionless even in its inculpations, so far-reaching in its views, it must everywhere be recognized as a speech which no other man could have made." Benjamin Brown French, a prominent Washington figure (former Clerk of the U.S. House of Representatives and the Commissioner of Public Buildings in D.C.), noted in his journal that he was in "the vast galleries of the Senate" ("hundreds who came to listen had to go away"), and opined that "It was a great speech. Let the *N.Y. Herald* and other papers of that *genius* say what they please against it—I say it was a great speech, and will *tell*." *Witness to the Young Republic: A Yankee's Journal, 1828-1870*, pp. 320-21 (Donald Cole & John McDonough eds.) (University Press of New England 1989).

9. Harold Holzer, *Lincoln at Cooper Union: The Speech That Made Abraham Lincoln President*, pp. 153-70 (Simon & Schuster 2004); C. Evan Stewart, "Lincoln in the Second Circuit," *Federal Bar Council Quarterly* (November 2011).

Joseph Medill, the *Chicago Press and Tribune's* Washington correspondent, wrote that Lincoln's "speech has created a sensation through the eastern states such as few speeches have ever done.... The signs now are, that if Seward is not nominated, Lincoln will be." That coverage prompted Seward to call on Medill and berate the journalist for having "gone back on him—and preferring that 'prairie statesman,' as he called Lincoln. . . . He dismissed me from his presence saying that thereafter he and I would no longer be friends." Sidney Blumenthal, *All the Powers of Earth*, p. 538 (Simon & Schuster 2019).

10. Blumenthal, supra note 9, p. 525.

CHAPTER II

The Republican National Convention

The Democratic National Convention—held at the end of April in Charleston, South Carolina—was an unmitigated disaster for that party. Southern delegates walked out in protest against Illinois Senator Stephen Douglas's candidacy; ultimately, a divided party put forward two candidates: the Northern wing, Douglas; and the Southern wing, President James Buchanan's Vice President, John Breckinridge (from Kentucky). This turn of events made the Republican nominee seem even more likely to win.[1]

The Republican Convention commenced in Chicago on May 16, Seward's fifty-ninth birthday, in a building newly constructed for the event called the Wigwam. Seward was back at this home in Auburn,

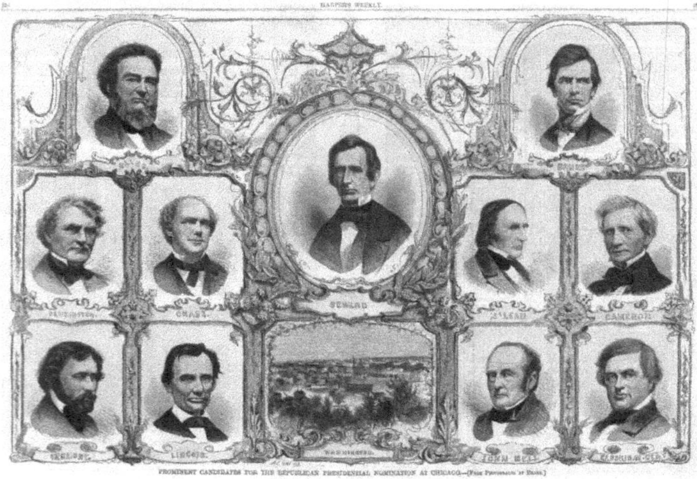

The Leading Republication Presidential Candidates in 1860
(Harper's Weekly, May 12, 1860)
(author's collection)

New York, trusting to Thurlow Weed and his lieutenants to ensure his nomination. Neighbors had moved Auburn's brass cannon next to the Seward home; it was to be fired upon news of his nomination.[2] And that made sense given that Seward was the party's presumptive nominee.[3]

The Wigwam was a gaslit, wooden firetrap (as all Chicago later proved to be); and it was filled to the rafters, not only with 465 delegates (from 24 states and three territories), but also with thousands of boisterous supporters for the home-town favorite, Abraham Lincoln—their counterfeit tickets had been distributed by Lincoln's campaign managers, depriving many Seward supporters (the "Irrepressibles") of their preapproved seats. And it was not only the Wigwam that was overstuffed, so too were the local hotels—where much of the political horsetrading took place over the next three days.[4]

Besides the location bias working against Seward, concern about carrying three states not won in 1856—Indiana, Illinois, and especially Pennsylvania (with its 27 Electoral College votes)—played a critical role. And this concern was manifested in two ways. The first was whether Seward—given his "irrepressible conflict" speech—was too "radical" to win key swing voters in those states. Unfortunately for Lincoln, the 1858 "House Divided" speech he gave in his Senate race against Stephen Douglas put him in the same "radical" boat on slavery as Seward's.[5]

The second manifestation was more important at both a practical and tactical political level. In 1856, the American Party had vied with the Republicans for dominance to oppose the Democrats. Led by former President Millard Fillmore, the party had done well, especially with two groups of voters—former

Whigs (who could not (yet) bring themselves to vote Republican), and anti-immigrant nativists, more commonly known as "Know Nothings."[6] While the electoral strength of the Know Nothings had reached its apex in the mid-1850s, it was still a very potent voting bloc in 1860 and the Republicans were determined to "fuse" those voters into their party (the two parties' 1856 vote totals nearly exceeded the Democrats in these three states).[7]

Here, the differences between Seward and Lincoln were profound. Seward, as Governor of New York, had publicly welcomed immigrants and, in particular, had taken affirmative steps to assist Irish Catholics (especially in the area of parochial schools). As such, nativists had a strong and well-established antipathy toward Seward.[8] Lincoln, on the other hand, while he had *privately* denounced the Know Nothing party,[9] he had taken no public position, having a large number of friends and political allies who were current or former members of that movement—people Lincoln wanted to "fuse" into the Republican Party.[10] This public versus private delineation proved to be a vital factor in strengthening Lincoln's position in those three states, all of which had well-documented nativist political strength.[11]

Another factor hurting Seward's candidacy was his former friend and political ally, Horace Greeley. Greeley,

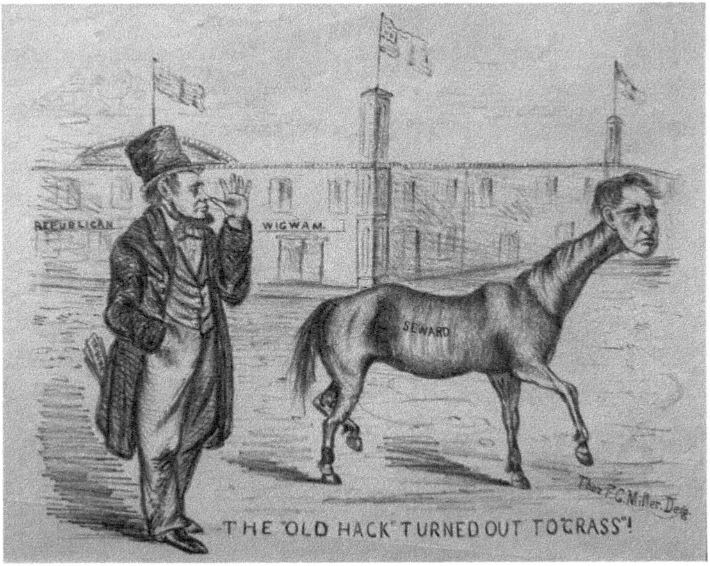

The "Old Hack" Tuned Out to "Grass"!
(1860 drawing by Thomas F.G. Miller)
(author's collection)

the editor of the powerful *New York Tribune,* had a (non-public) falling out with Seward and Weed when they declined to support him in 1855 for New York Lieutenant Governor. Heading to the convention as a Bates delegate from Oregon, Greeley had met with Weed in Albany and implied that he would nonetheless end up backing Seward.[12] At the Convention, however, Greeley (who everyone assumed was still close to Seward and Weed) "devoted every hour ... to the most steady and relentless prosecution of the main business which took him thither—the defeat of Governor Seward."[13]

Lincoln's (and his campaign manager's) strategy of trying to be the "available" candidate—everyone's second choice (and, being less well-known, not being directly attacked head-on by the leading candidates) also played a role.[14] Not only did it help to keep him from frontal assaults, it also exposed the weaknesses of other front-runners. For example, with respect to Bates (a former Know Nothing), the prominent (and growing) group of Republican German-Americans (allied to Lincoln) expressly resolved not to support a Bates-led ticket.[15] Chase had other problems: although nationally prominent, the Ohio delegation was not unanimous in support of his candidacy; that doomed his efforts to gain support in other states.[16]

All of the foregoing may, or may not, have been enough to stop Seward's nomination. What indisputably *did* stop it was the political skill (which included outright bribery) of Lincoln's campaign manager, David B. Davis. Davis—an old colleague of Lincoln's from their days of riding the Illinois legal circuit[17]—not only worked himself and his lieutenants mercilessly, he also decided to out-Weed Weed.

When one of Davis's men wired Lincoln, "A pledge or two may be necessary when the push comes," Lincoln wired back: "I authorize no bargains, and will be bound by none," Davis just ignored Lincoln's wire ("Lincoln aint here").[18] To win over the Indiana delegation, Caleb Smith (the chairman) was promised a cabinet post (ultimately he became the Secretary of the Interior); and William Dole was promised the Commissioner of Indian Affairs.[19] Then late on May 17—the first two days of the Convention having gone well for the Seward forces—Davis played his ace card to get the Pennsylvania delegation. Joseph Medill (of the *Chicago Press & Tribune*) confronted Davis just after his midnight meeting with the delegation:

> Medill: "How will they vote?"
> Davis: "Darned if we haven't got them,"
> Medill: "How did you get them?"
> Davis: "By paying their price." [Senator Cameron to become Secretary of the Treasury]
> Medill: "Great Heavens! Give Cameron the Treasury Department? What will be left?"
> Davis: "Oh, What's the difference? We are after a bigger thing than that; we want the Presidency, and the Treasury is not a great stake to pay for it."[20]

On May 18, the balloting began.[21] After the first go-round, Seward was ahead with 173½ votes (about 60 short of victory), but Lincoln had 102 (including the entire Indiana delegation, as well as votes from delegates from Southern states where Republicans had *no* chance in November—e.g., Lincoln got 14 delegates from Virginia). On the second ballot Seward's total rose to 184½; but Cameron honored his deal with Davis and 48 (out of

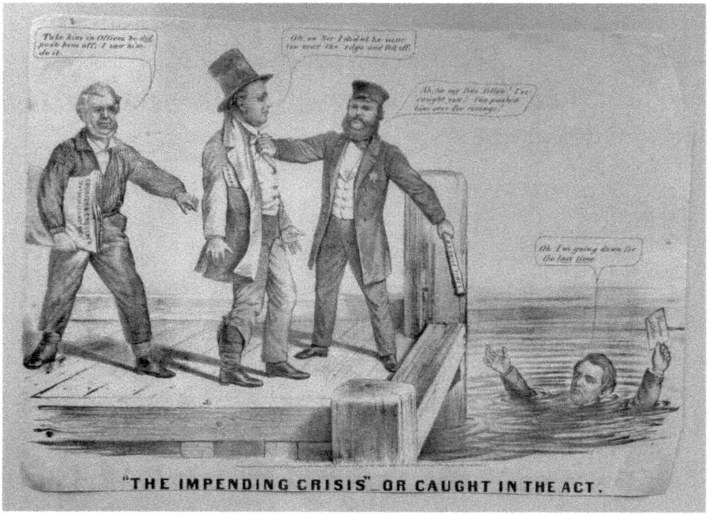

"The Impending Crisis" or Caught in the Act
(1860 drawing by Louis Maurer; published by Courier & Ives)
(author's collection)

54) Pennsylvania's delegates switched from favorite-son Cameron to Lincoln, which brought him to 181.[22] With that momentum, the third ballot saw Lincoln surge to 231½, 1½ votes short of the nomination. Ohio, with a not-so-gentle push, then changed four votes to Lincoln—and (in the words of Murat Halstead) "The deed was done.").[23] Thereupon, William Evarts (head of the New York delegation) rose and moved to make the nomination unanimous.[24]

Back in Auburn, a friend brought a telegram to Seward that read "Lincoln nominated on the third ballot." Seward, without any emotion, said: "Well, Mr. Lincoln will be elected and he has some of the qualities to make a good president."[25] Later, the brass cannon was moved back to the town square in Auburn.[26]

Notes

1. Besides Murat Halstead's excellent accounts of the Democratic conventions (see infra note 2), see Michael Holt's *The Election of 1860: A Campaign Fraught with Consequences*, pp. 50-66 & 115-33 (University Press of Kansas 2017); see also Glyndon Van Deusen, *William Henry Seward*, p. 220 (Oxford University Press 1967); Walter Stahr, *Seward: Lincoln's Indispensable Man*, p. 185 (Simon & Schuster 2012); *The Letters of Stephen A. Douglas*, pp. 492-96 (Robert Johannsen ed.) (University of Illinois Press 1961). Curiously, Seward

(at least initially) did not see the Democratic division as politically helpful. In a May 4, 1860, letter to his wife he wrote:

> Just at the moment when one party, pressed by the other, is seeking to disavow the cardinal article of the uncompromising antagonism between freedom and slavery in the country, the party that denies it is riven asunder by the very antagonism which it had disputed. I am on the lookout now for the next pretext of demoralization among Republicans.

Frederick W. Seward, *Seward at Washington: 1846-61*, p. 448 (Derby and Miller 1891).

2. There are two excellent accounts of the 1860 Republican Convention: a contemporaneous account by journalist Murat Halstead (see William Hesseltine's *Three Against Lincoln: Murat Halstead Reports the Caucuses of 1860* (Louisiana States University Press 1960)), and Sidney Blumenthal's 2019 account (*All the Powers of Earth* (Simon & Schuster)). See also Edward Achorn's "The Lincoln Miracle" (Atlantic Monthly 2023); Urman Ray's *The Convention That Nominated Lincoln* (University of Chicago Press 1916); Gary Ecelbarger's *The Great Comeback: How Abraham Lincoln Beat the Odds to Win the 1860 Republican Nomination* (St. Murha's 2013).

3. The *Providence Post* reported that "the nomination belongs to him"; and the *Washington Evening Star* wrote that Seward would be the nominee since he was the "great representative man" of the party. Stahr, supra note 1, p. 185. Even a Democratic Party's newspaper acknowledged his status. See *Atlas and Argus* (Albany, NY, May 19, 1860) ("We have recognized the genius and leadership of the man."). Horace Greely, editor of the *New York Tribune* (a former close ally and now bitter foe of Seward's—as explained above in the text)

wired back to the *Tribune* staff on May 17: "My conclusion, from all I can gather tonight, is that the opposition to Governor Seward cannot concentrate on any candidate, and that he will be nominated." Hesseltine, supra note 2, p. 161; Blumenthal, supra note 2, p. 591; Van Deusen, supra note 1, p. 223.

4. See Halstead's description of the Tremont House, with 1,500 people "stowed away," in Hesseltine, supra note 2, pp. 141-42.

5. In an April 24, 1860, letter, Illinois Senator Lyman Trumbull reported to Lincoln that, when he urged Republican politicians in Washington to support Lincoln over Seward: "I am almost always met with the remark, 'if you are going to nominate a man of that stamp, why not take Seward.' There seems to be a disposition in the public mind to associate you together, from the fact, I suppose, that you have both given expression to a similar statement in regard to the ultimate extinction of slavery." Abraham Lincoln Papers (Library of Congress).

Lincoln tried to finesse this problem by stressing to supporters that, while he and Seward were on the same page on the subject of "irrepressible conflict," he (Lincoln) had never endorsed Seward's "A Higher Law" position. Holt, *The Election of 1860*, supra note 1, pp. 101-02.

6. See Tyler Anbinder, *Nativism and Slavery: The Northern Know Nothings and the Politics of the 1850s* (Oxford University Press 1992); John Mulkern, *The Know-Nothing Party in Massachusetts: The Rise and Fall of a People's Movement* (Northeastern University Press 1990); Ray Billington, *The Protestant Crusades 1800-1860: A Study of the Origins of American Nativism* (Quadrangle 1964); Luke Ritter, *Inventing America's First Immigration Crisis: Political Nativism in the Antebellum West* (Fordham University Press 2021); Eugene Roseboom, "Salmon P. Chase and the Know Nothings," *Mississippi Valley*

Historical Review (1938-39); William Gienapp, "The Transformation of Cincinnati Politics" (Seminar Paper, Yale 1969); Sister M. Evangeline Thomas, "Nativism in the Old Northwest, 1850-1860" (Washington D.C. 1936); Ira Leonard & Robert Parmet, "American Nativism, 1830-1860" (New York 1978); Henry Carmon & Rienhard Luthin, "Some Aspects of the Know-Nothing Movement Reconsidered," *South Atlantic Quarterly* (1940); William Bean, "The Aspect of Know Nothingism—The Immigrant and Slavery," *South Atlantic Quarterly* (1924); Stephen Maizlish, "The Meaning of Nativism and the Crisis of the Antebellum North," *Essays on American Antebellum Politics 1846-1860* (Texas A&M University Press 1982) (Stephen Maizlish & John Kushma eds.); William Gienapp, "Politics Seem to Enter into Everything: Political Culture in the North 1840-1860," [see Maizlish, just above]; Joel Silbey, "The Surge of Republican Power: Partisan Antipathy, American Social Conflict, and the Coming of the Civil War" [see Maizlish, just above]; William Gienapp, *The Origins of the Republican Party 1852-1856* (Oxford University Press 1987); Michael Holt, *The Election of 1860* (supra note 1), *The Rise and Fall of the American Whig Party: Jacksonian Politics and the Onset of the Civil War* (Oxford University Press 2003), *Political Parties and American Political Development from the Age of Jackson to the Age of Lincoln* (Louisiana State University Press 1992), *The Political Crisis of the 1850s* (Wiley 1978); Jean Baker, "Ambivalent Americans: The Know-Nothing Party in Maryland" (Johns Hopkins University Press 1977); William Gienapp, "Who Voted for Lincoln?" *Abraham Lincoln and the American Political Tradition* (University of Massachusetts Press 1986) (John Thomas, ed.).

7. See the comparative analyses of the 1856, 1858-59, and 1860 election results in Holt, *The Election of 1860*, supra note 1, Appendix A.

8. Stahr, supra note 1, p. 191. Emblematic of the harsh antipathy by nativists toward Seward on this score is a letter Thurlow Weed received from one Know-Nothing, urging him to drop Seward as a presidential candidate: "[There is] widespread and deep prejudice against Seward on account of his action, as governor, on the public schools ... [whereby immigrants could be taught by] teachers speaking the same language ... and professing the same faith.... The prejudice [against him] pervades the entire Protestant church.... It is strongest with the clergy; but it is showed more or less by the great body of the laity, even outside the council of the Know Nothings ... while with the Americans, it is rankest—deepest—most bitter." O.B. Vienz November 27, 1858, letter to Weed (Weed Papers, Library of Congress). See also Janet Coryell, *Neither Heroine nor Fool: Anna Ella Carroll of Maryland*, p. 41 (Kent State University Press 1990). Recognizing this problem, Seward had consulted with Weed in April 1860 about the wisdom of having a well-known Know-Nothing, Congressman Henry Winter Davis (of Maryland), be considered for the vice presidential slot. Stahr, supra note 1, p. 184; Van Deusen, supra note 1, p. 222; John M. Taylor, *William Henry Seward: Lincoln's Right Hand*, pp. 116-17 (HarperCollins 1991). In 1859, Jefferson Davis had predicted that disputes between "Black Republicans" and the "Americans" might "prevent the nomination of Seward." Davis June 4, 1859, letter to J.L.M. Curry (Democratic Congressman, Alabama) *Jefferson Davis: The Essential Writings*, pp. 161-62 (William Cooper, ed.) (Random House 2003).

9. See Roy Basler (ed.), *The Collected Works of Abraham Lincoln* (Rutgers University Press 1953-55); Volume 2, pp. 321-23 (Lincoln letter to Joshua Speed, August 24, 1855) ("I am not a Know Nothing. That is certain. How could I be? How can anyone who abhors the oppression of negroes, be in favor of degrading classes of

white people? Our progress in degeneracy appears to me to be pretty rapid. As a nation, we began by declaring that 'all men are created equal, *except negroes*.' When the Know-Nothings get control, it will read 'all men are created except negroes, *and foreigners, and catholics*.' When it comes to this I should prefer emigrating to some country where they make no pretense of loving liberty—to Russia, for instance, where despotism can be take pure, and without the base allow of hypocracy[sic].").

For a detailed explication of Lincoln's careful dealings with the Know Nothing party in Illinois (and key individuals therein) during the 1850s, see Harold Holzer, *Brought Forth on this Continent: Abraham Lincoln and American Immigration*, pp. 69-82 (Dutton 2024); see also Stahr, supra note 1, pp. 191-92; Holt, *The Election of 1860*, supra note 1, p. 24. For an analysis of how Lincoln (and his political advisors) "fused" with mid-western Know Nothing voters in the 1860 election, see William Harris, *Lincoln and the Border State: Preserving the Union*, pp. 12-18 (University Press of Kansas 2011).

10. Lincoln, moreover, had a growing alliance with many Midwestern German-Americans (which included an ownership interest in a politically oriented German newspaper). See Holzer, supra note 9, pp. 114-15, 127-45.

11. See John Senning, "The Know-Nothing Movement in Illinois 1854-1856," *Journal of the Illinois State Historical Society* (April 1914); Stephen Hansen & Paul Nygard, "Stephen A. Douglas, the Know-Nothings, and the Democratic Party in Illinois," *Illinois State Historical Journal* (Summer 1994); William Gienapp, "Nebraska, Nativism, and Rum: The Failure of Fusion in Pennsylvania, 1854," *The Philadelphia Magazine of History and Biography* (*PMHB*) (1985); James Huston, "The Demise of the Pennsylvania American Party, 1854-1858," *PMHB* (1985); William Gudelunas, "Nativism and the

Demise of Schuylkill County Whiggery: Anti-Slavery or Anti-Catholicism," *Pennsylvania History* (1978); Frank Gerrity, "The Disruption of the Philadelphia Whigocracy: Joseph R. Chandler, Anti-Catholicism, and the Congressional Elections of 1854," *PHMB* (1987); Gerald Eggert, "'Seeing Sam': The Know Nothing Episode in Harrisburg," *PHMB* (1987); William Gienapp, "Nativism and the Creation of a Republican Majority in the North Before the Civil War," *Journal of American History* (1985); Bruce Levine, "'The Vital Element of the Republican Party': Antislavery, Nativism, and Abraham Lincoln," *Journal of the Civil War Era* (2011); Robert Sullivan, "John Mitchell and His Critics: Transatlantic Abolition and the Irish American Response to Slavery in the 1850s," *Civil War History* (2025). See also Harris, supra note 9, pp. 5-18.

According to one of Greeley's lieutenants at the *New York Tribune*, Republican candidates for Governor in both Pennsylvania and Indiana believed that Know-Nothing antipathy for Seward's record as New York's Governor (especially in funding Catholic schools) would defeat them in their races. Abram J. Dittenhoefer, *How We Elected Lincoln and Men of His Time*, pp. 21-22 (Harper Brothers 1916); see also A.K. McClure, *Abraham Lincoln & Men of War-Times*, pp. 33-35 (Times Publishing 1892); Blumenthal, supra note 2, pp. 581-82; Hesseltine, supra note 2, p. 149.

On May 15, 1860, and May 16, 1860, the *Chicago Press and Tribune* ran two lead articles that stressed Lincoln's ability to carry the three states because "he is acceptable to the mass of the American Party" ("The Winning Man—Abraham Lincoln" & "The Doubtful States"). Blumenthal, supra note 2, p. 578.

12. Blumenthal, supra note 2, p. 581; Lawrence Denton, *William Henry Seward and the Secession Crisis*, p. 14 (McFarland & Company 2009).

13. Blumenthal, supra note 2, p. 581 (quoting Henry Raymond, editor of the *New York Times*); see also Van Deusen, supra note 1, pp. 225-26.

14. Holt, *The Election of 1860*, supra note 1, pp. 88-114. As Lincoln said: "I suppose I am not the first choice of a very great many.... Our policy, then, is to give no offense to others—leave them in a mood to come to us, if they shall be compelled to give up their first love." Mark Neely, *The Last Hope on Earth*, p. 219 (Harvard University Press 1993).

15. Blumenthal, supra note 2, pp. 578-80 & 590-91; Hesseltine, supra note 2, p. 144.

16. Blumenthal, supra note 2, pp. 571-72; Hesseltine, supra note 2, p. 144.

17. Lincoln ultimately appointed Davis to the U.S. Supreme Court. See C. Evan Stewart, *The Worst Supreme Court Decisions, Ever! (And Related Tales)* (Chapter XVIII) (Twelve Tables Press 2024).

18. Taylor, supra note 8, p. 7. Interestingly, that did not stop the Lincoln contingent from flirting with taking the number two spot if Seward ultimately prevailed. Id. p. 7; see also Blumenthal, supra note 2, p. 585.

19. Blumenthal, supra note 2, p. 583.

20. Stefan Lorant, *The Glorious Burden*, p. 242 (Harper & Row 1976); Blumenthal, supra note 2, pp. 582-83; Stahr, supra note 1, p. 190; Denton, supra note 12, p. 15. Cameron ultimately became Secretary of War.

It is highly ironic that Davis and his colleagues proved to out-corrupt Weed, who had a public reputation for frequently crossing the line. It appears that Weed (and his lieutenants) were overconfident, believing that advocacy of Seward's record and offers of money—alone—would do the trick in Chicago; they were wrong.

Blumenthal, supra note 2, pp. 584-89; Stahr, supra note 1, p. 190; Van Deusen, supra note 1, pp. 223-24; Denton, supra note 12, pp. 17-18; Taylor, supra note 8, pp. 7-10. Years later Cameron reportedly claimed that Weed's failure to meet with him in Harrisburg, Pennsylvania, prior to the convention caused Cameron to repudiate his proffer of support to Seward the prior year. Glydon Van Deusen, *Thurlow Weed: Wizard of the Lobby*, pp. 248-49 (Little Brown and Company 1947).

21. Seward's conventional managers wired him that morning: "Everything indicates your nomination today sure." Van Deusen, supra note 20, p. 224.

22. One of my ancestors, who had been a Fillmore elector in 1856, cast his first ballot in Chicago for Cameron and then switched to Lincoln on the second and third ballots (as directed by Cameron).

23. Joseph Medill (of the *Chicago Press and Tribune*), seated next to the Chairman of the Ohio delegation (David Carter), whispered in Carter's ear: "If you can throw the Ohio delegation to Lincoln, Chase can have anything he wants." Carter then switched four votes from Chase to Lincoln, and Lincoln was nominated. Blumenthal, supra note 2, p. 594. [Chase later became the Secretary of the Treasury in Lincolns first term; and thereafter was nominated (and became) Chief Justice of the U.S. Supreme Court.]

24. Evarts (a Seward protégé) would later serve as President Johnson's lead lawyer in his 1868 impeachment trial in the U.S. Senate, and thereafter serve as U.S. Attorney General, New York Senator, and Secretary of State. See C. Evan Stewart, *Law in American History (And in Mine)* (Chapter XXXI) (Twelve Tables Press 2025). For Evarts's motion, see F. Seward, supra note 1, p. 451; J. Hampden Dougherty, *William M. Evarts: Lawyer and Statesman*, pp. 8-9 (Kessinger Publishing Rare Reprints 1901).

25. Stahr, supra note 1, pp. 388-89; Van Deusen, supra note 20, p. 225; Taylor, supra note 8, p. 9. Maine Senator Hannibal Hamlin was nominated on the second ballot to be Lincoln's running mate. As Murat Halstead reported: "it was stated that Mr. Hamlin was a good friend of Mr. Seward. He was geographically distant from Lincoln, and was once a Democrat." Hesseltine, supra note 2, p. 174.

26. Weed was disconsolate; he broke down and wept at his failure to deliver the nomination to Seward. Blumenthal, supra note 2, pp. 594-95; Taylor, supra note 8, p. 9; Denton, supra note 12, p. 19 (as did Weed's lieutenants and the mass of Seward's supporters: the "Irrepressibles"). Later that day Seward wrote to Weed:

> You have my unbounded gratitude for this last, as for the whole life of efforts in my behalf. I wish that I was sure that your sense of the disappointment is as light as my own. It ought to be equally so, for we have been equally thoughtful and zealous, for friends, party, and country, and I know not what has been left undone that could have been done, or done that ought to be regretted.

F. Seward, supra note 1, p. 453; Thurlow W. Barnes, *Memoir of Thurlow Weed*, p. 270 (Houghton Mifflin 1884).

As reported by Murat Halstead:

> The fact of the Convention was the defeat of Seward rather than the nomination of Lincoln. It was the triumph of a presumption of availability over pre-eminence of intellect and unrivaled fame—a success of the ruder qualities of manhood and the more homely attributes of popularity over the arts of a consummate politician and the splendor of accomplished statesmanship.

Hesseltine, supra note 2, pp. 176-77.

CHAPTER III

Seward's Role in the 1860 Campaign

While outwardly stoic, Seward was devastated by his loss.[1] His immediate reaction was to end his public career at the conclusion of his Senate term (in early 1861) and retire to Auburn; he had no intention of campaigning for the Republican ticket, nor did he want to be in a new administration's cabinet.[2]

Nonetheless, Seward rebounded quickly (at least publicly). On May 19, he wrote an editorial for the local paper endorsing the party's ticket: "No truer or firmer defenders of the Republican faith could have been found in the Union than the distinguished and esteemed citizens on whom the honors of the nomination have fallen."[3] Two days later, in responding to a lengthy letter from New York's Republican Central Committee about the outcome of the Chicago convention, Seward wrote:

> I find in the resolutions of the Convention a platform as satisfactory to me as if it had been framed with my own hands; and in the candidates adopted by it, eminent and able Republicans with whom I have cordially co-operated in maintaining the principles embodied in that

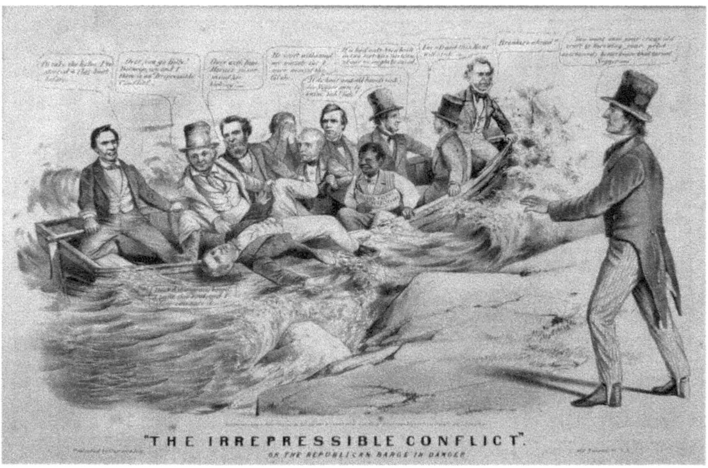

"The Irrepressible Conflict" or the Republican Barge in Danger (1860 drawing by Louis Maurer; published by Courier & Ives) (author's collection)

> excellent creed. I cheerfully give them a sincere and earnest support.[4]

At the end of the month Seward made his way back to Washington for the new session of the Thirty-Sixth Congress. In route, he stopped in Albany to meet with Thurlow Weed. After the convention Weed had visited Abraham Lincoln before returning home. The dictator was impressed with the party's candidate, finding that Lincoln not only understood the state-by-state complexities of the upcoming election, but was also a person with "so much good sense, such intuitive knowledge of human nature, and such familiarity with the virtues and infirmities of politicians."[5] Seward's political mentor was thus planning to work hard in the lead-up to the November election (with the message to Seward that he should do likewise).

When he walked onto the Senate floor in Washington, Seward was greeted "kindly" by (the duplicitous) Simon Cameron and "cordially and manfully" by a few Republican Senators (including Charles Sumner), with others of his party showing a "consciousness of embarrassment." More interesting were the "frank, open, [and] sympathizing words" expressed by some of his long-time Southern Democratic political opponents, including Jefferson Davis.[6]

During the Congressional session a number of Seward's political friends and allies pressed home the same theme expressed by Weed. Most important were the words and advice from his good friend Congressman Charles Francis Adams, son of Seward's political hero, John Quincy Adams.[7] Adams told Seward that "his services are more necessary to the course than they ever were [and] your own reputation will gain more of permancy from the becoming manner with which you meet this disappointment than it would from all the brilliancy of the highest success."[8]

After the Congressional session adjourned, the divided Democratic Party met twice in Baltimore. On June 18, the Northern section nominated Lincoln's former Senate opponent Stephen Douglas for President; and on June 28, the Southern section nominated President James Buchanan's vice president, John Breckinridge (of Kentucky), for the presidency. A fourth party—the Constitutional Union Party (mostly consisting of conservative, border state men (former Whigs)—had previously met in May and nominated Tennessee slaveholder John Bell for president. As a result, the 1860 campaign would be a unique contest in American history, with essentially two different races: a Northern contest—Lincoln vs. Douglas; and a Southern contest—Breckinridge vs. Bell. To many observers it appeared that perhaps no candidate would receive a majority in the Electoral College, and the presidency would have to be resolved in the U.S. House of Representatives.[9]

While this political picture was coming into focus, Seward began to think about what role, in fact, he might play in the campaign. As always, he sought the wise counsel of Thurlow Weed. On June 26 he wrote Weed:

> If I can rightly, and to the satisfaction of my friends, remain at rest, I want to do so. I am content to quit with the political world, when it proposed to quit with me. But I am not insensitive to the claims of a million of friends, nor indifferent to the opinion of mankind. All that seems clear to me, just now, is that it would not be wise to rush in at the beginning of the canvass, and so seem, most falsely, to fear that I shall be forgotten. Later in the canvas, it may be seen that I am wanted for the public interest. Of all this I want to talk with you quietly.[10]

Even before meeting with Weed, Seward accepted a speaking engagement in Michigan. Thereafter, on July 6 he wrote to Weed that "some part of, perhaps a considerate one, of the responsibility of electing [Lincoln] rests on us." As such, he planned (in the future) to "go to Chicago or any of the 'pivotal' states which may demand it."[11]

But first Seward traveled to Windsor, Vermont, to visit William Evarts at his summer home. Also present were other Seward political allies, including Weed and James Watson Webb, the editor of the *Morning Courier & New York Enquirer*.[12] As Seward had indicated in his earlier letter to Weed, these days were devoted to planning what Seward would do leading up to the election (and how to finance his efforts).

From Windsor, Seward took a picturesque train ride through New Hampshire (Bellows Falls, Keene, and Dover) ultimately arriving in Bangor, Maine. There, despite a heavy downpour, he was met by a crowd of several thousand. At each stop along the way, Seward was pressed to speak. In Bangor, he explained that he had come at the invitation of his friend Congressman Israel Washburn (new Republican candidate for Governor): Maine was clearly "on the side of freedom and free labor," and thus Maine's citizens should vote "for the able and upright statesman of the West, Abraham Lincoln of Illinois and your own talented and able citizen [vice presidential nominee, Hannibal Hamlin]."[13]

After meeting with Washburn in Portland, Maine, Seward headed south to Boston (staying at various towns on the way and making brief speeches at each). Among the thousands meeting the train in Boston were Seward's friend Congressman Adams and his eldest son, Charles Francis Adams Jr. Besides giving a political speech invoking his hero, John Quincy Adams, who he likened to Lincoln in their support for the freedom of man, Seward spent a day at the Adams's family home in Quincy. During his stay he lobbied (ultimately successfully) for Adams and his son to join him on his

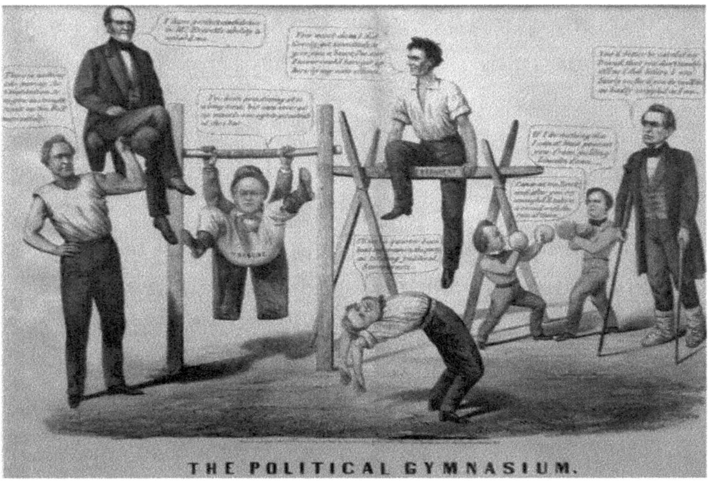

The Political Gymnasium
(1860 drawing Louis Maurer; published by Courier & Ives)
(author's collection)

upcoming (extensive) campaign travels throughout the North.[14]

On September 1, the Seward party left Auburn by train. Initially, his daughter, Fanny, and some family friends were on board; at various stops along the way some political cronies also joined the train (and before long the two Adams had gotten on board as well).

Seward's messages at each train stop varied. At one he used humor. Asking the assembled group why they had come, he queried: "Is it a question? I have no party to sell. What do I hear? The Whig Party? Going, going, gone. The American Party? Going, going, gone.... This train, too. Going, going, gone."[15] At another he pooh-poohed the Fire-Eaters' threat(s):

> The slave power ... rails now with a feeble voice, instead of thundering as it did in our ears for twenty or thirty years past. With a feeble and muttering voice they cry out that they will tear the Union to pieces. They complain that if we will not surrender our principles, and our system, and our right, being a majority to rule, and if we will not accept their system and such rules as they will give us, they will go out of the Union. Who's afraid? Nobody's afraid![16]

From Niagara the Seward party (via Canada) moved on to Detroit, where he was met by thousands of people, caravans, rockets, and (as was the case virtually everywhere on the trip) a large group of "Wide Awakes." The Wide Awakes (originally formed by 12 young men in Hartford, Connecticut, on March 3, 1860) was a paramilitary-looking assemblage that led Republican torchlight parades; it exponentially spread throughout the Northern states, and had a galvanizing effect on large crowds (and, because of their youth, the Wide Awakes especially attracted young male voters to the Republican cause).[17] It was to that part of his audience Seward made a direct appeal:

> Today the young men of the United States are for the first time on the side of freedom against slavery. Go then and do your work. Put this great cause into the keeping of your great, honest, worthy leader, Abraham Lincoln. Believe me sincere, when I say, that if it had devolved upon me to select from all the men in the United States a man whom I should confide the standard of their cause—which is the object for which I have lived and labored, and for which I would die—that man would be Abraham Lincoln.[18]

After stopping at other cities across the state of Michigan the Seward entourage moved on to Wisconsin. In the capital (Madison), he found numerous people yelling out from the crowd identifying their original New York roots. To those voices Seward replied: "Why, I thought I was midway between the lakes and the Mississippi, but I find I am at home, among old neighbors and friends."[19]

Reaching the Mississippi River, the group got on a steamboat and headed toward St. Paul, Minnesota. Various towns along the way required Seward to stop and speak; and he was met at each with "enthusiastic salutations."[20] Upon reaching St. Paul (in spite of the rain and mud), it "seemed to be a gathering of the Whole State."[21] To the assembled thousands, part of Seward's address seemed to foreshadow one of his greatest public accomplishments:

> Standing here and looking far off into the North-west, I see the Russian as he busily occupies himself in establishing sea-ports and towns, and fortifications on the verge of this continent as the outposts of St. Petersburg, and I can say: 'Go on, and build up your outposts all along the coast, up even to the Arctic Ocean—they will yet become the outposts of

> my own country—monuments of the civilization of the United States in the North-west."[22]

From Minnesota the Seward party got back on a steamboat and headed south to Iowa, ultimately arriving in Dubuque, where Seward spoke to an audience of several thousand people. While (again) stressing that a Republican victory posed no threat to the Southern states and their "peculiar institution,"[23] Seward made clear the choice voters faced:

> The time comes at last when Nature unerringly vindicates every right, and punishes every wrong in the actions of men or States. She comes then in terror, in revolution, in anarchy, in chaos. You will let this Government and the nation slide down still further the smooth declivity of national vice if you choose. Nature will bring it back again in due time with convalescence which will wake the sighs and groans of the civilized world.[24]

Heading further south to Kansas (where Seward had received "so many earnest invitations"), the traveling party had first to come into Missouri—a slave state where the Republicans stood no chance. In the town of

Chillicothe a curious crowd of "pro-slavery men" assembled to hear him speak. From the platform of his railroad car, Seward told the crowd that Bell, Douglas, and Breckinridge were all "good personal friends of mine, of whom I always speak well." Seeing a wide variety of political support in evidence, he "in a good humoured strain" observed that since they could not seem to agree on one of their candidates, they should perhaps "agree on *my* candidate, Abraham Lincoln."[25]

Kansas, at this point, was not yet a state (and thus could offer no votes), but given its importance in giving rise to the Republican Party—and its ongoing symbolism to the North of the aggressiveness of the "Slave-Power"—Seward wanted to visit the territory.[26] Hailed as "the Representative of Kansas, in the Senate of the United States" and "the Defender of Kansas and of Freedom!," Seward declared that the people of Kansas are "the most intelligent, and the bravest, and the most virtuous people of the United States." They had "take[n] the banner of human freedom, when it is trailed in the dust, by the Government of their choice, and can and does raise it aloft, and protect it, and bear it to success and honor."[27]

Next, via St. Louis, Seward's party traveled to Illinois for the big finale. In route to Chicago, the train first stopped in Springfield so Lincoln could meet with his new champion.[28] From Charles Francis Adams Jr.'s perspective, Lincoln was "very awkward in manner; as if he felt out of place, and had a realizing sense that properly the positions should be reversed."[29] From the rear of the railroad car, Seward promised the crowd (and Lincoln) that the "State of New York will give a generous and cheerful, and effective support to your neighbor, Abraham Lincoln."[30]

For weeks Seward's Chicago appearance had been promoted by the Chicago press; as a result, the largest crowd in Illinois political history (over 200,000 people) turned out to see and hear Seward speak on October 2.[31] His speech was "long and elaborate" ("the National Idea"), but its political message was direct and pointed: the other three candidates (and parties) offered either no solution, or demonstrably flawed ones, regarding how to deal with the existential conflict facing America—freedom versus slavery. Only the Republican Party had the ideology and the leadership to address that conflict and ensure that America could become "a new and great empire."[32] According to one account, when Seward finished "[t]he ovation did not end until late at night; and then, with a serenade, and a huge procession of 'Wide Awakes.'"[33]

Chicago turned out to be not quite the finale, for as Seward's train headed eastward, he was importuned to speak to large audiences in Cleveland and Buffalo, as well as to crowds in smaller towns along the way.[34] By October 6, Seward reached Auburn, where he was greeted by his hometown friends as a returning, conquering hero.

Although exhausted, Seward could not rest for long; he soon learned that carrying New York State was no longer a sure thing. Republican leaders had been buoyed by gubernatorial victories in the October state elections that preceded presidential voting in November (especially in the key states of Pennsylvania and Indiana).[35] But now the three parties opposing the Republican Party—in a desperate (but ingenious) way to stop its electoral success—engaged in realpolitik: they agreed to join forces and put forward a "Fusion" ticket of New York State electors under a "Union" label. Funded heavily by Wall Street (which had deep ties to Southern commerce and greatly feared the economic fallout of secession, especially by the "Cotton States"), the "Union" electors might well carry New York State—which would deprive Lincoln of an Electoral College majority, throwing the race into the U.S. House of Representatives (where the Republican ticket would likely lose).[36]

On October 25, Weed asked Seward to come to (heavily Democratic) New York City and give a "soothing speech … [to show] that it is the business of Republicans and the mission of the Republican party to preserve the Union."[37] The exhausted (and sick) Seward agreed.

On November 2 (four days before the voting), Seward appeared before an overflow crowd at the Palace Garden. He delivered the "soothing speech" asked for by Weed: a Republican administration would "leave things to go on just exactly as they have gone on hitherto"; slavery in the Southern states would "be gradually, peacefully circumscribed and limited hereafter, as it has been hitherto"[38]; and freedom in the territories would be protected "just exactly as it is now."[39]

While the speech may have been "soothing," the crowd's reaction was not: "benches were smashed in the crush"; "Seward's speech was interrupted repeatedly by cheers and applause, and at its conclusion there was a deafening ovation." That was followed by "Old Abe's Choir" singing "Ain't We Glad Abe's Going to the White House," which was itself followed up with:

> In '64 with peace secured
> We will have our William Seward.[40]

On November 6, 1860, the nation voted. In every state in which Seward had campaigned (except

Missouri), the Republican ticket prevailed. In New York City, the Fusion Party outpolled the Republican Party; but thanks to upstate voting, Lincoln's statewide margin was almost 60,000 votes.[41] And with New York State's electoral votes safely in hand, Abraham Lincoln was now president-elect.

Notes

1. Walter Stahr, *Seward: Lincoln's Indispensable Man,* p. 189 (Simon & Schuster 2012); John M. Taylor, *William Henry Seward: Lincoln's Right Hand,* p. 119 (HarperCollins 1991); Glyndon Van Deusen, *William Henry Seward,* pp. 228-29 (Oxford University Press 1967); Lawrence Denton, *William Henry Seward and the Secession Crisis,* p. 22(McFarland & Company 2009). In later years Seward would demonstrate different reactions to this defeat. To a family physician, he acknowledged his political weakness in Pennsylvania: "without her we could not carry the election; hence I was not an available man. Mr. Lincoln [on the other hand] possessed all the necessary qualifications to represent our party; and being comparatively unknown, had not to contend with the animosities generally marshalled against a leader." Stahr, supra this note, pp. 192-93. To a congressman arguing that denying a diplomatic assignment to Carl Schurz (a prominent German-American) would be "a severe disappointment to a good many people," Seward angrily rebuked him: "Disappointment! You speak to me of disappointment. To me, who was justly entitled to the Republican nomination for the presidency, and who had to stand aside and see it given to a little Illinois lawyer! You speak to me of

disappointment!" Sidney Blumenthal, *All the Powers of Earth*, p. 595 (Simon & Schuster 2019).

2. Stahr, supra note 1, p. 194; Taylor, supra note 1, pp. 119-20. Seward's wife, Frances, was very pleased about this development. [Mrs. Seward was not fond of Washington and was a very infrequent visitor there, both pre and post 1861.]

3. *Auburn Daily Advertiser* (May 19, 1960).

4. Frederick W. Seward, *Seward at Washington: 1846-61*, p. 454 (Derby and Miller 1891). Seward's entire reply was printed on the front page of the *New York Times* (May 25, 1860).

5. Thurlow W. Barnes, *Memoir of Thurlow Weed*, pp. 602-03 (Houghton Mifflin 1884); Stahr, supra note 1, p. 195.

6. Seward May 30, 1860, letter to Francis Seward (Seward Papers, University of Rochester); F. Seward, supra note 4, pp. 455-56; Taylor, supra note 1, p. 120; Stahr, supra note 1, p. 195.

7. In 1848 Seward delivered two separate (and famous) eulogies in honor of his hero, J.Q. Adams. See Stahr, supra note 1, pp. 105-09.

8. Adams May 22, 1860, letter to Seward (Seward Papers, University of Rochester); Stahr, supra note 1, p. 196; Van Deuson, supra note 1, pp. 230-31; Denton, supra note 1, p. 23. Besides the flowery language, Adams also told Seward that the untested Lincoln needed not only his electoral help but also would need Seward's experience and skill in running the national government: "the cabinet of Mr. Lincoln cannot be left to itself, or to feeble men, without shipwreck." C.F. Adams Diary (June 21, 1860) (Massachusetts Historical Society); Stahr, supra note 1, p. 196.

Henry Adams, the Congressman's younger son, has provided the most famous description of Seward's appearance: "A slouching, slender figure; a head like a wise macaw; a beaked nose; shaggy eyebrows; unorderly hair and clothes; hoarse voice; offhand manner; free talk, and perpetual cigar ... a type in one way simple because it was only double—political and personal; but complex because the political had become nature, and no one could tell which was the mask and which the features." Henry Adams, *The Education of Henry Adams*, p. 104 (Houghton Mifflin Sentry Edition 1961). For other depictions of Seward, compare Denton, supra note 1, p. 25 (a "young, handsome 'John F. Kennedy' of his generation") with William Russell, *My Diary North and South*, p. 40 (Eugene Berwanger ed.) (McGraw Hill 1988) ("A well-formed and large head is placed on a long, slender neck, and projects over the chest in an argumentative kind of way, as if the keen eyes were seeking for an adversary; the mouth is remarkedly flexible, large but well formed, the nose prominent and aquiline, the eyes secret, but penetrating, and lively with humor of some kind twinkling about them; the brow bold and broad, but remarkable elevated; the white hair silvery and fine—a subtle, quick man, rejoicing in power, given to perorate and to oracular utterances, fond of badinage, bursting with the importance of state mysteries, and with the dignity of directing policy of the greatest country—as all Americans think—in the world.").

9. See Michael Holt, *The Election of 1860: A Campaign Fraught with Consequences*, pp. 134-66 (University Press of Kansas 2017). For an excellent analysis of the electoral threat posed by the Constitutional Union Party, see id. at pp. 67-87.

10. F. Seward, supra note 4, p. 459; Barnes, supra note 5, pp. 297-98.

11. Seward July 6, 1860, letter to Weed (Weed Papers, University of Rochester); Stahr, supra note 1, p. 197. Seward, by this point, had also agreed to speak in Minnesota; he had also been asked to speak in Illinois on August 8 (a request seconded by Lincoln), but

it was turned down because of a conflict. Van Deusen, supra note 1, p. 231.

12. Stahr, supra note 1, p. 197; Van Deusen, supra note 1, p. 231.

13. Stahr, supra note 1, p. 197; *Bangor Daily Whig & Courier* (August 13, 1860).

14. Stahr, supra note 1, pp. 199-200; Van Deusen, supra note 1, pp. 231-32; Taylor, supra note 1, p. 121; F. Seward, supra note 4, pp. 459-60.

15. Stahr, supra note 1, p. 201.

16. *The Works of William H. Seward* (ed. George Baker), Vol. 4, p. 344 (Houghton Mifflin 1884); David Potter, *The Impending Crisis*, p. 432 (Harper & Row 1976); Taylor, supra note 1, p. 121; Van Deusen, supra note 1, p. 233; Stahr, supra note 1, p. 204. Even James Buchanan (in 1856) had said: "We have so often called 'Wolf,' that now, when the wolf is at the door, it is difficult to make the people believe it." *The Works of James Buchanan* (John Moore ed.), Vol. 2, p. 180 (J.B. Lippincott 1908-1911).

17. Holt, supra note 9, pp. 138-40; F. Seward, supra note 4, pp. 461-70; Stahr, supra note 1, pp. 202-06. In the Southern states the paramilitary nature of this fast-growing group of Republican activists was viewed as a "knife to our throats." Id. In the North some Douglas supporters established "The Chloroformers"—groups designed to put the Wide Awakes to sleep. Stefan Lorant, *The Glorious Burden*, p. 246 (Harper & Row 1976); Holt, supra note 9, p. 140.

18. F. Steward, supra note 4, p. 246.

19. F. Seward, supra note 4, p. 463.

20. F. Seward, supra note 4, p. 464.

21. F. Seward, supra note 4, p. 464.

22. F. Seward, supra note 4, p. 464; see also Taylor, supra note 1, p. 123; Stahr, supra note 1, p. 204.

23. In Detroit Seward also tried to address Southern racial fears about a Republican administration:

> The great fact is now fully realized that the African race here is a foreign and feeble element, … incapable of assimilation.… It is a pitiful exotic unnecessarily transported into our fields, and which it is unprofitable to cultivate at the cost of the desolation of the native vineyard.

Taylor, supra note 1, p. 122.

24. F. Seward, supra note 4, p. 465; Stahr, supra note 1, p. 204. At one point during the campaign trip one of Seward's companions remarked: "You are doing more for Lincoln's election than any one hundred men in the United States." Stahr, supra note 1, p. 209.

Also during this period young Adams wrote in his diary: "I never could understand where, when or how [Seward] … prepared the really remarkable speeches he delivered in rapid succession." Stahr, supra note 1, pp. 205 n.47, 594 n.44; Taylor, supra note 1, p. 122.

25. F. Seward, supra note 4, pp. 465-66.

26. The attempt to impose slavery in Kansas had led to widespread violence and acts of terrorism that shocked Northern voters. See Holt, supra note 9, pp. 6-20. For the best study of the importance of "Bleeding Kansas" to the rise of the Republican Party, see William Gienapp's *Origins of the Republican Party, 1852-1856* (Oxford University Press 1987); see also James McPherson, *Battle Cry of Freedom: The Civil War Era*, pp. 145-69 (Oxford University Press 1988). For the Buchanan administration's politically inept handling of the Kansas issue, see *James Buchanan and the Political Crisis of the 1850s*

(Michael Birkner ed.) (Susquehanna University Press 1996); *James Buchanan and the Coming of the Civil War* (John Quist & Michael Birkner eds.) (University of Florida Press 2013).

27. F. Seward, supra note 4, pp. 466-68; Stahr, supra note 1, p. 205.

28. The two men had met once before—in September 1848; Seward and Lincoln had both spoken at a Whig campaign rally for Zachary Taylor in Boston. The following night they shared the same bedroom in Worcester, Massachusetts, where they talked late into the night about the "slavery question." C. Evan Stewart, *Law in American History (And in Mine)* (Chapter XXVII) (Twelve Tables Press 2025); Stahr, supra note 1, pp. 110-11, 119.

29. Charles Francis Adams Jr., *Autobiography*, pp. 64-65 (Houghton Mifflin 1916); Van Deusen, supra note 1, p. 233.

30. F. Seward, supra note 4, pp. 468-69; see also Stahr, supra note 1, pp. 205-06 (Seward "promised that the Republicans would have a majority of 60,000 votes in New York"). Michael Burlingame (who clearly is no fan of Seward) portrays Seward's visit to Springfield, as well as his entire trip canvassing support for Lincoln, in a (to put it mildly) negative light. *Abraham Lincoln: A Life*, Volume I, pp. 653-56 (Johns Hopkins University Press 2009).

31. Denton, supra note 1, p. 23; Stahr, supra note 1, p. 206; F. Seward, supra note 4, pp. 169-70.

32. *The New York Times* (October 3 & 6, 1860); F. Seward, supra note 4, pp. 469-70; Stahr, supra note 1, p. 206.

33. F. Seward, supra note 4, p. 470.

34. On the trip east one night, Seward's train (at rest) had an unusual visitor: Senator Stephan Douglas, who was frantically touring the country (in violation of the then prevailing political custom that presidential candidates did not campaign for themselves).

Douglas, whiskey bottle in hand, burst into Seward's berth and demanded that Seward "come out and speak to the boys!" Seward demurred: "I can't go out. I'm sleepy." Ultimately, the well-lubricated candidate left Seward alone. Charles Francis Adams Jr., supra note 29, pp. 65-69; Taylor, supra note 1, p. 123; Stahr, supra note 1, pp. 206-07.

35. Lincoln, in fact, wrote to Seward that these results "surpassed all expectation, even the most extravagant.... It now really looks as if the Government is about to fall into our hands." Lincoln letter of October 12, 1860, to Seward. Roy Basler (ed.), *The Collected Works of Abraham Lincoln*, Volume 4, pp. 126-27 (Rutgers University Press 1953-55).

36. See Holt, supra note 9, pp. 152-53, 171, 173; F. Seward, supra note 4, pp. 472-73; Stahr, supra note 1, pp. 207-08; Van Deusen, supra note 1, pp. 234-34. For analyses of the Republican campaign to woo nativist voters and prevent "fusion" efforts in the key swing states of Indiana, Illinois, and Pennsylvania, see Burlingame, supra note 30, Volume I, pp. 659-64, 670-71, 682-83; William Harris, *Lincoln and the Border State: Preserving the Union*, pp. 16-18 (University Press of Kansas 2011). Initially, Douglas was opposed to fusion. Douglas July 4, 1860, letter to N. Paschall ("An amalgation ticket with the bolters would disgust the people and give every Northern State to Lincoln."), *The Letters of Stephen A. Douglas*, p. 497 (Robert Johannsen ed.) (University of Illinois Press 1961).

Complicating the Republicans' task in New York was a proposed constitutional amendment on the ballot to allow free Blacks to vote (doing away with a significant property requirement). Democrats campaigned against the unpopular ("universal negro suffrage") proposal, linking it to the Republican Party. See Phyllis Field, *The*

Politics of Race in New York: The Struggle for Black Suffrage in the Civil War Era, pp. 114-46 (Cornell University Press 1982).

37. Tweed letter of October 25, 1860 to Seward (Seward Papers, University of Rochester).

38. The Republican plan to limit slavery "hereafter" is well explained in James Oakes's *The Scorpion's Sting: Antislavery and the Coming of the Civil War* (W.W. Norton 2014).

39. F. Seward, supra note 4, pp. 473-74; Stahr, supra note 1, p. 208. On November 3, Weed wrote to Lincoln about the lavish spending of the fusion leaders. But he concluded: while "[s]ome of our friends are nervous, ... I have no fear of the result in this State." Barnes, supra note 5, pp. 350-51.

40. Van Deusen, supra note 1, p. 235. See F. Seward, supra note 4, pp. 474-75 for Seward's speech in Auburn on election eve.

41. See Holt, supra note 9, Appendix A (In New York State: Republicans: 362,646 (53.6%); Fusion 314,282 (46.4%)). As Holt makes clear (see id. p. 173), because of the fusion efforts in New York (and other states) the actual vote totals of Douglas, Bell, and Breckinridge are impossible to ascertain with certainty.

The proposed constitutional amendment to allow universal suffrage in New York State lost by 140,000 votes. Holt, supra note 9, p. 159.

Chapter IV

November 1860—The Aftermath of Lincoln's Election

The night of the election brought a report that both of South Carolina's Senators—in response to Lincoln's victory—had resigned from the Senate. Days later the state itself was poised to secede from the Union (with a December 20 date set for a convention); and four other states from the Deep South soon thereafter established dates for their own secession conventions.[1]

One Alabama newspaper declared that Lincoln's election "shows the North [intends] to free the negroes and enforce amalgamation between them and the children of the poor men of the South"; and one North Carolina newspaper prophesized that "if we submit now to Lincoln's election your homes will be visited by one of the most fearful and horrible butcheries that has cursed the face of the globe"; while a Fire-Eater from Georgia wailed that if Georgia remained in a nation "ruled by Lincoln and his crew . . . in TEN years or less our CHILDREN will be the *slaves* of negroes."[2]

Lincoln was a longtime skeptic of secession threats. Before the election he told a visitor to Springfield: "I don't think they will. . . . I will convince them that I do not wish to interfere with them in any way, but protect them in everything that they are entitled to."[3] Lincoln also drew optimism based on the election results in the South, because Stephen Douglas and John Bell—who both opposed secession—outpolled John Breckinridge by 110,000 votes (with Bell carrying both Virginia and Tennessee, and nearly winning North Carolina and Maryland; Douglas and Bell together won over 70 percent of the vote totals in Missouri).[4] Following the advice recommended by Republican newspaper editors, as well as political advisors, Lincoln decided to engage in "masterly inactivity"—to not say anything in public, or write any on-the-record letters, expressing himself vis-à-vis the Southern threat of dis-Union—in the hope that the crisis would abate with the passage of time (as cooler heads in the South asserted themselves).[5]

Seward, on the other hand, quickly came to the realization that the secession threat was real. And although he had planned to remain at his home in

Auburn, New York, through December, he decided that he needed to be in Washington instead[6]—to "save the Union in my own way."[7]

But first Seward went to confer with Thurlow Weed, initially in Albany (on November 16) and later in New York City (on November 29). Those dates are significant because Weed issued editorials in the *Albany Evening Journal* on November 19 and November 30. By those editorials Weed argued that the Republican victory had rendered slavery's expansion into the territories academic (at best), since the new Republican administration would be in charge of them (thus ensuring freedom therein and not requiring specific legislation); and as an olive branch to the South, he advocated that Congress reinstate the Missouri Compromise (nullified by the Kansas-Nebraska Act of 1854),[8] which would bar slavery in the territories above 36°30', while allowing slavery below that line—making clear, however, that (in his view) this concession would have no practical effect since the latter (Southern) area was completely unsuitable for chattel slavery. Weed also proposed that a national convention at some future date be convened so that North and South "might this bring their respective griefs, claims, and reforms to a common arbitrament, to meet discuss, and determine upon a future."[9]

With these trial balloons aloft, Seward arrived back in Washington, just as November came to a close; his monumental task of saving the Union his "own way" would face many severe challenges (from friends and foes).[10]

Notes

1. An excellent overview of the immediate aftermath of the election can be found in James McPherson's *Battle Cry of Freedom: The Civil War Era*, pp. 234-75 (Oxford University Press 1988).

2. Donald Reynolds, *Editors Make War: Southern Newspapers in the Secession Crisis*, pp. 125-25 & 141 (Southern Illinois University Press 2006); Michael Johnson, *Toward a Patriarchal Republic: The Secession of Georgia*, pp. 47-48 (Louisiana State University Press 1977).

For a comprehensive collective-biography of the leading Southern secessionists, see Eric Walther's *The Fire-Eaters* (Louisiana State University Press 1992). For an excellent biography of one of the most consequential Southern politicians who advocated secession, see Eric Walther's *William Lowndes Yancey and the Coming of the Civil War* (University of North Carolina Press 2006). An invaluable source of information on this subject can also be found in the three-volume diary of the man who fired the first shot on Fort Sumter, thereby starting the Civil War: *The Diary of Edmund Ruffin* (William Scarborough ed.) (Louisiana State University Press 1972-1989). For the Secession Commissioners' role in galvanizing support in the Cotton States for leaving the Union, see Charles Drew, *Apostles of*

Disunion (University Press of Virginia 2001). See also "The Politics of Slavery Affirmed: The South and the Secession Crisis" in Michael Cooper's *Approaching Civil War and Southern History*, pp. 56-74 (Louisiana State University Press 2019); William Freehling, *The Road to Disunion: Secessionists Triumphant, 1859-1861* (Oxford University Press 2007).

3. Parmenas Taylor Turnley, *Reminiscences of Parmenas Taylor Turnley, from the Cradle to Three Score and Ten*, p. 10 (Donohue & Henneberry 1892). To another visitor Lincoln got a little hot under the collar. Calling the alarmists "liars and knaves," Lincoln exclaimed, "This is the same old trick by which the South breaks down every Northern victory." John Nicolas & John Hay, *Abraham Lincoln: A History*, Volume 3, pp. 280-81 (The Century Co. 1890); Michael Burlingame, *Abraham Lincoln: A Life*, Volume I, pp. 698-99 (Johns Hopkins University Press 2009).

4. Burlingame, supra note 3, Volume I, pp. 692-03. For the exact vote totals in all states for the 1860 election, see Michael Holt, *The Election of 1860: A Campaign Fraught with Consequences*, Appendix A (University Press of Kansas 2017). Both Weed and Seward similarly analyzed the 1860 vote vis-à-vis anti-secession sentiment:

> It was an indisputable fact that the vote count for Douglas, numbering 1,365,976, and that cast for Bell, numbering 590,631, and the vote for Breckinridge in the free states, numbering 284,422, making a total of 2,241,029, was unanimously in favor of a peaceful and reasonable settlement of all difficulties with any of the Southern States.... Thus the voice of the people of the country ... was overwhelmingly in favor of conciliation.

James Rhodes, *History of the United States from 1850 to 1877*, Volume 3, p. 261 (Macmillan 1910); see also Lawrence Denton, *William Henry Seward and the Secession Crisis*, p. 73 (McFarland & Company 2009).

But, as we will see, their analysis led them to chart a different course from Lincoln's (i.e., a strategy to appeal to those anti-secessionist voters by seeking some common ground(s) with them and thus keeping them in the Union).

5. Burlingame, supra note 3, Volume I, pp. 100-02. When asked to reassure southerners who honestly believed they were in real danger because of his victory, Lincoln famously replied: "there are no such men." *Recollected Words of Abraham Lincoln*, p. 341 (Don Fehrenbacher & Virginia Fehrenbacher, eds.) (Stanford University Press 1996). Furthermore, and as Daniel Crofts has written: "Lincoln had a fatalistic sense that any reassurances from him [in November and December] 'would do no good' and might do 'positive harm.' Secessionists, thinking a new statement evidence of his 'timidity,' would clamor all the louder." As such, Lincoln communicated his view on these critical issues by "private and confidential" letters. *Reluctant Confederates: Upper South Unionists in the Secession Crisis*, pp. 224-25 (University of North Carolina Press 1989); see also Lincoln December 15, 1860, letter to Gilmer (*The Collected Works of Abraham Lincoln*, Volume 4, pp. 151-52 (Roy Basler ed.) (Rutgers University Press 1953-55)). Harold Holzer, *Lincoln, President-Elect: Abraham Lincoln and the Great Secession Winter 1860-1861*, pp. 114-47 (Simon & Schuster 2008), devoted an entire chapter to Lincoln's decision; the title thereof reveals Holzer's view of that decision ("A Masterly Inactivity"). Burlingame, on the other hand, concluded that Lincoln's decision to be publicly silent "may have been a mistake." (supra note 3, p. 702).

Lincoln's "private and confidential" letters displayed no "timidity," especially with respect to the issue of compromise. After the House of Representatives established a "Committee of Thirty-Three" in early December 1860, in an attempt to prevent dis-Union, Lincoln wrote to Congressman William Kellogg (Illinois's representative on the Committee): There could be no "compromise in regard to the *extension* of slavery. The instant you do, they have us under again, all our labor is lost.... Douglas is sure to be again trying to bring in his 'Pop.' Sov." Have none of it. *The tug has to come and better now than later*." Lincoln December 11, 1860, letter to Kellogg (Basler, Volume 4, p. 150) (emphasis added). Two days later Lincoln sent a similar message to Illinois Congressman E.B. Washburne: "[Do not] entertain [] propositions for compromise of any sort, on 'slavery extension.' ... On that point hold firm, *as with a chain of steel*." Lincoln December 13, 1860, letter to Washburne (Basler, Volume 4, p. 151) (emphasis added). See also Burlingame, supra note 3, Volume I, pp. 708-09; Holzer, supra note 5, pp. 155-60.

At the same time Lincoln was assuring correspondents that—to conciliate the South—he would strongly enforce the Fugitive Slave Act. See, e.g., Lincoln December 11, 1860, letter to Kellogg (cited above); Burlingame, supra note 3, Volume I, p. 209 ("He assured a Kentucky Democrat that the Fugitive Slave Law 'will be better administered under my Administration than it ever has been under that of my predecessors.'").

6. Seward November 18, 1860, letter to Weed (quoted in Frederick W. Seward, *Seward at Washington: 1846-61*, p. 478 (Derby and Miller 1891)); see also Glyndon Van Deusen, *William Henry Seward*, p. 238 (Oxford University Press 1967); Seward November 15, 1860, letter to Weed (Weed Papers, University of Rochester).

7. Seward actually said these words on January 25, 1861. See James Adams Lawrence Diary (Massachusetts Historical Society); Walter Stahr, *Seward: Lincoln's Indispensable Man*, pp. 211, 232 (Simon & Schuster 2012).

8. Three years later the U.S. Supreme Court, in *Dred Scott v. John F.A. Sanford*, 60 U.S. (19 How.) 393 (1857), had also held the 1820 law establishing the Missouri Compromise to be unconstitutional. See C. Evan Stewart, *The Worst Supreme Court Decisions, Ever! (And Related Tales)* (Chapter I) (Twelve Tables Press 2024).

9. *Albany Evening Journal* (November 19 and November 30, 1860); F. Seward, supra note 6, p. 479; Crofts, supra note 5, p. 219. Horace Greeley, in the *New York Tribune*, suggested that the North "let the erring sisters depart in peace" (November 9 and November 27, 1860); Seward's ally, Henry Raymond of the *New York Times*, advocated revising the Fugitive Slave Law and repealing the Northern States' "personal liberty laws" (which had been enacted to neuter enforcement of the Fugitive Slave Law) (November 14 and November 19 and November 21, 1960).

Seward's only public comment in November 1860 came in a speech he gave to a celebrating group of "Wide Awakes" who came to serenade him at his home in Auburn. While well pleased that the flawed national policy of 40 years had been "retraced, reconsidered, reversed, and renounced," Seward urged them to be magnanimous in victory and "show the greater virtue of moderation in triumph." As for those defeated in the election, they "are not, never can be, never must be, enemies, or even adversaries. We are all fellow-citizens, Americans, brethren." F. Seward, supra note 6, p. 476; Stahr, supra note 7, p. 211.

10. At the same time Lincoln was telling Republican colleagues not to entertain notices of compromise (see supra note 5),

as Michael Holt observed: "Other Republicans [i.e., Seward and Weed] had a far more astute appreciation of the seriousness of the secessionist threat. They agreed that the party could benefit, rather than suffer, from making concessions by forming a winning political alliance with the southern opponents of secession who were pleading for evidence that the Republicans would not subject white Southerners either to abolition or degrading political subjugation." Holt, supra note 4, p. 182. Holt went on to cite (in detail) Weed's December 10, 1860, letter to Seward's fellow New York Republican Senator, Preston King: with Lincoln's election "[t]he fight is over … the issues of the late campaign are obsolete." Because the new administration would appoint all territorial governors, there could be no slavery extension. "My dear old friend, the sooner you put on your thinking cap and impress your colleagues with a sense of the dangers, the more you will rejoice for the rest of your life." Id. at p. 188.

Chapter V

December 1860—Seward Goes to Work

In a December 1 letter to his wife, Seward wrote "Nothing new to-day":

> The ultra-Southern men *mean* to break up the Union, not really for the grievances of which they complain, but from cherished disloyalty and ambition. The President, and all Union men there are alarmed and despondent. The Republicans who come here are ignorant of the real design or danger. I begin to see my way through, without sacrifice of principle. But I talk very little, and nothing in detail.[1]

But Seward was misleading his wife. Thurlow Weed's November editorials had enraged many of his Republican colleagues as an abandonment of Republican principles;[2] and given his closeness to Weed, they attributed the editorials to Seward. Attempting to neutralize the political fallout (and keep his options open), Seward was forced to quickly (and repeatedly) deny that he had anything to do with what Weed had expressed, that they did not express his views, and that he had not yet formed his views. He went so far as to plant a story in the *New York Tribune* in which he (writing in the third person) wrote: "He is in no manner or form responsible for the various suggestions recently put forward in various newspapers, which have been supposed to reflect his views, and was not consulted concerning, or in any way privy to, their publication."[3]

Seward's protestations were, to put it bluntly, not true. While his public dissembling(s) may have placated the political world, no historians who have studied this period believe that Weed acted without Seward's express and explicit agreement.[4] Indeed, as Seward once said: "Seward is Weed and Weed is Seward. What I do, Weed approves. What he says, I endorse. We are one."[5]

And although Seward publicly claimed *not* to have formed any views, in fact he had. Recognizing that the "Cotton States" were lost to the Union (at least for the time being), he believed that the best hope was to do everything possible to keep the Upper South in the

Union; and if he was successful in achieving that goal, economic and other pressures would likely cause the seceding states to come back into the fold.[6]

At this same moment a weak (and terrified) lame-duck president issued his final address to Congress. Blaming the secession crisis on the "incessant and violent agitation of the slavery question throughout the North for the past quarter of a century," James Buchanan bravely pronounced that secession was unconstitutional, *but* that the federal government was powerless to stop any state that seceded.[7] Lincoln was incensed at Buchanan's address;[8] Seward's take was somewhat different: "The Message … shows conclusively that it is the duty of the President to execute the laws—unless someone opposes him—and that no State has a right to go out of the Union—unless it wants to."[9]

By letters dated December 8, 1860, Lincoln formally asked Seward to be Secretary of State in the new administration. The actual details may be lost to history,[10] but the best reconstruction of events is as follows. Leaving the Capitol on December 12 with his friend Senator Hannibal Hamlin (soon to be vice president), Seward was handed two letters. The first was a brief formal offer. The second (labeled "private and confidential") directly addressed the public rumors that any cabinet offer to Seward would be merely pro forma: "I have said nothing to justify these rumors.... [Rather] it has been my purpose, from the day of the nomination at Chicago, to assign you, by your leave, this place in this administration.... [Y]our position in the public eye, your integrity, ability, learning, and great experience, all combine to render it an appointment preeminently fit to be made."[11] Lincoln's keen insight into how to manipulate even someone of Seward's ego proved spot on. According to Hamlin, Seward's face became "pale with excitement" as he read the second letter and he exclaimed: "This is remarkable, Mr. Hamlin. I will consider the matter, and, in accordance with Mr. Lincoln's request give him my decision at the earliest practicable moment."[12]

Remarkable or not, after consulting with Weed, Seward wrote Lincoln on December 16 that he had asked Weed to visit Lincoln to discuss "the condition and the prospect of public affairs; and he will be able to inform you of my prescient unsettled view of the subject upon which you so kindly wrote me a few days ago."[13] By such a meeting Weed could sound out Lincoln not only on Seward's expected role in the cabinet but also the president-elect's intentions vis-à-vis other cabinet positions (and attempt to influence them).[14]

December 20, 1860

December 20 was a critical day in the Secession Winter for two reasons. First, it was the day the South Carolina Convention unanimously voted to secede from the Union. It was also the day Thurlow Weed sat down for a lengthy meeting with Abraham Lincoln in Springfield, Illinois. Unfortunately, the meeting did not start on a positive note.

On December 17, just before leaving Albany, Weed had published his most expansive editorial, advocating conciliatory measures to avoid a constitutional crisis; again he called for the reinstatement of the Missouri Compromise, also writing that the *Albany Evening Journal* was "*almost* prepared to say, that Territories may be safely left to take care of themselves; and that, when they contain a Population which … entitles them to a Representative in Congress, they may come into the Union with State Governments of their own framing."[15]

As Weed later recalled, Lincoln began by telling Weed that his editorial was "a heavy broadside": "You have opened your fire at a critical moment, aiming at friends and foes alike. It will do some good or much mischief."[16] Making clear that he would not agree to a compromise based on an expansion of slavery ("hold firm, as with a chain of steel"), Lincoln gave Weed a single-page document containing three resolutions that he asked that Seward submit to Congress:

> Resolved:
>
> That the fugitive slave clause of the Constitution ought to be enforced by a law of Congress, with efficient provisions for that object, not obliging private persons to assisting in its execution, but punishing all who resist it, and with the usual safeguards to liberty; securing free men against being surrendered as slaves—
>
> That all state laws, if there be such, really, or apparently, in conflict with such law of Congress, out to be repealed; and no opposition to the execution of such law of Congress ought to be made—
>
> That the Federal Union must be preserved.[17]

Lincoln then turned to the subject that Weed was more focused on: the potential make-up of Lincoln's cabinet. Weed had hoped to persuade the president-elect to pick men not only favorable to Seward politically but also those more open to conciliation efforts to the Upper South. This lobbying effort was not a great success. Instead of Charles Francis Adams (proposed by Weed as a representative of New England), Lincoln said he was disposed to appoint Connecticut publisher Gideon Welles (a former Democrat); he also intended to appoint Salmon Chase for the Treasury post (Chase was also a former Democrat; he was also publicly against any and all compromises).[18]

Weed then pressed to have some Southerners in the cabinet. When Lincoln questioned whether any could "be trusted," Weed replied: "the men I have in mind can always be relied on." Asked to name them, Weed gave Lincoln four—former Whigs with strong Union ties; the only one that Lincoln showed interest in was Congressman John Gilmer of North Carolina.[19] Lincoln told Weed he would write to Gilmer, and also authorized Weed to meet with the Gilmer to discuss a possible appointment.[20]

Lincoln then brought up some Southern names of his own: "Judge [Montgomery] Blair has been suggested." Weed was incredulous: "I object to Judge Blair because he represents nobody, he has no following [except his famous father Francis (political advisor to Andrew Jackson)], and because his appointment would be obnoxious to the Union men of Maryland; and that, as I believe, while he can look to Maryland, he actually resides in the District of Columbia."[21] Undeterred,

Lincoln said: "Very well, I will now give you the name of a gentleman who not only resides in a slave state, but who is emphatically a representative man. What objection do you to Edward Bates of Missouri?" To that name Weed answered: "None, not a shadow or a shade of an objection. That is a selection, as Webster might have said, 'eminently fit to be made.'"[22]

As the six-hour session wound down, a downcast Weed observed that there would be too few former Whigs in Lincoln's cabinet. To that Lincoln countered: "You seem to forget that *I* expect to be there, and counting me as one, you can see how nicely the cabinet would be balanced and ballasted."[23]

December 18, right before the major events of December 20, the Senate had appointed the "Committee of Thirteen," to address possible measures to avoid the constitutional crisis (the House had earlier constituted a similar group on December 4—the "Committee of Thirty-Three).[24] The Senate group was comprised of that body's most important members, including Seward, Stephen Douglas, Jefferson Davis, and (the heir to Henry Clay's Kentucky Senate seat) John Crittenden. The first order of business of the Committee of Thirteen was to consider the Crittenden Compromise—a plan he had made public two days before.

Crittenden's plan was a series of amendments to the Constitution:

- a guarantee of slavery in the states against future interference by the federal government;
- prohibition of slavery in territories north of 36°30', but slavery protected in territories south of that line "now held, *or hereafter acquired*" (emphasis added);
- barring Congress from abolishing slavery on any federal property within the slave states;
- barring Congress from abolishing slavery in the District of Columbia (i) without the consent of its residents, *and* (ii) unless it had first been abolished by both Maryland and Virginia;
- barring Congress from interfering with the interstate slave trade;
- compensating slave owners prevented from recovering fugitive slaves in Northern states;
- making these amendments permanent and not subject to future revision or nullification.[25]

But before Seward could turn his attention to the Senate Committee and the Crittenden Compromise, he had to meet with Weed upon his return from Springfield. On a train from Syracuse to Albany, Weed gave Seward a rundown of his disappointing meeting with Lincoln.[26]

Seward then continued on to New York City. Checking in at the Astor Hotel at 11 p.m., he found that the New England Society were celebrating "Fore-Fathers' Day." It was a group consisting of many political and personal friends, so Seward could not say no to their importunings to attend and speak to them. He was surprisingly upbeat and optimistic. The Union was like any family where, on occasion, family members "become discontented and wish to withdraw for a while." But if a foreign nation were to descend "upon the City of New York tomorrow … the hills of South Carolina would pour forth their population to the rescue." And if South Carolina were to be attacked, "I know who would go to their rescue." He concluded:

> I believe the cause of secession was as strong, on the night of November 6, when the President and Vice President were elected—and who were unacceptable to the slave states—as it has been at any time. Some fifty days have

> now passed; and I believe that every day the sun has set since that time, it has set upon mollified passions and prejudices; and if you will only await the time, sixty more suns will shed a light and illuminate a more cheerful atmosphere.[27]

Arriving in Washington on December 24, Seward met with the four other Republican members of the Committee (and later the whole Committee). As he wrote to his wife that night, the Committee had come "to no compromise; and we shall not. We shall, therefore, see the fuller development of the secession movement."[28] What he did not report to his wife was that Seward had repackaged what Lincoln had given Weed into a different formulation:

- the Constitution should be amended so that Congress could never interfere with slavery in the slave states;
- the Fugitive Slave Law should be amended to allow for a jury trial;
- the states should repeal any laws inconsistent with the Constitution and existing federal laws [i.e., the Northern personal liberty laws].

When the full Committee met, all five Republicans voted against the restoration of the Missouri Compromise [the "or hereafter acquired" language meant Cuba, and not even Seward could agree to that].[29] The Committee did approve Seward's first proposal (by an 11-to-2 vote), but the others received no affirmative support.[30]

The day after Christmas Seward wrote Lincoln a lengthy letter reporting on the deliberations of the Committee of Thirteen: "With the unanimous consent of our section, I offered three propositions which seemed to cover the ground of the suggestion made by you, through Mr. Weed, as I understood it." [Claiming not to have received the document Lincoln gave Weed until that morning], Seward further reported that Republican members of the Committee (together with Senators Lyman Trumbull and William Fessenden) had met at his home that night to consider whether "your written suggestions ... shall be offered." Seward wrote that the group concluded not to do so—"it would divide our friends, not only in the Committee but in Congress."

Seward then changed tack and told Lincoln "what I think of the *temper* of the *parties* of the *public* here." In his view, even with the restoration of the Missouri Compromise, all the Cotton States would still leave the Union. But:

> The action of the border States is uncertain. Sympathy there is strong with the Cotton States, while prudence and patriotism dictate adhesion to the Union. Nothing could *certainly* restrain them, but the adoption of Mr. Crittenden's compromise; and I do not see the slightest indication of its adoption, on the Republican side of Congress.[31]

The next day Major Robert Anderson moved his troops from the indefensible Fort Moultrie in Charleston, South Carolina, to the more defensible Fort Sumter; that caused President Buchanan's cabinet to collapse, with its Southern members bolting.

Seward wrote several letters to Lincoln the next day. First, he alerted him to the "fevered excitement here," suggesting that Lincoln come to Washington earlier than planned so he could get a better understanding of the mood of the U.S. Capitol. He also wrote to suggest additional Southern Unionists for Lincoln's cabinet. And, finally, he wrote:

> I have, after due reflection and with much self-distrust, concluded that if I should be nominated to the Senate for the office of Secretary of State, and the nomination should be

> confirmed, it would be my duty to accept the appointment.[32]

Seward was busy on other fronts as 1860 came to an end. On December 28, he met with James Orr, who had come to Washington to seek recognition of South Carolina as an independent country. Orr told Seward that Major Anderson's action was perceived in a number of Southern states as "unanswerable evidence" that the federal government planned "to coerce South Carolina." Using a technique he would perfect over the next several months, Seward agreed that Anderson's "movement was a most unfortunate one" and suggested that it might be possible to have Anderson evacuate Sumter and return to his prior (hard to defend) fort.[33]

And behind the scenes (in collaboration with his close friend and political ally, Charles Francis Adams) Seward was also helping to devise two alternatives to the Crittenden Compromise in the House of Representatives. The first became known as the "New Mexico Plan," whereby the large Western territory south of the Missouri Compromise line would be admitted into the Union as a state without regard to slavery (New Mexico had a slave code and 11 slaves within the territory—but most people believed it was inhospitable to plantation slavery), with the large territory north of 36°30' being free of slavery. A slightly different proposal—the so-called Border State Plan—would have forbidden Congress, as well as any territorial legislature, from enacting a law for or against slavery south of the Missouri Compromise line.[34] While there appeared to be some early optimism for some version of these compromise proposals—they in fact did divide the Upper South from the Lower South (and there was some possibility of passage, at least in the House of Representatives)[35]—what these proposals really accomplished was to buy time for Seward in the coming months of the New Year to try to hold the Upper South in the Union—at least until Lincoln could take office on March 4, 1961.[36]

Notes

1. Seward December 1, 1860, letter to Francis Seward (quoted in Frederick W. Seward, *Seward at Washington: 1846-61*, p. 478 (Derby and Miller 1891).

2. For a good sample of radical Republican reactions to Weed's trial balloons (as well as Lincoln's), see Michael Burlingame, *Abraham Lincoln: A Life*, Volume I, pp. 695-98 (Johns Hopkins University Press 2009).

3. *New York Tribune* (December 3 and December 5, 1860); Walter Stahr, *Seward: Lincoln's Indispensable Man*, p. 212 (Simon & Schuster 2012); Glyndon Van Deusen, *William Henry Seward*, p. 239 (Oxford University Press 1967).

4. See Frederic Bancroft, *The Life of William H. Seward,* Volume 2, pp. 26-29 (Harper & Row 1900) ("Weed and Seward were never in closer communication than during these months ... he and Seward were working together like the hand of one man"); Daniel Crofts, *Reluctant Confederates: Upper South Unionists in the Secession Crisis,* p. 219 (University of North Carolina Press 1989); Stahr, supra note 3, p. 212. See also Patrick Sowle's "The Conciliatory Republicans During the Winter of Secession" (Ph.D. dissertation, Duke University 1963).

5. Gideon Welles, *Lincoln and Seward,* p. 23 (Sheldon 1874). In letters to his wife, Seward was more candid: "You will see that Mr. Weed lets me out of responsibility for his well-intentioned, but rather impulsive movements" (December 2); "Mr. Weed's articles have brought perplexities about me which he, with all his astuteness, did not foresee" (December 4); and as to the *Tribune* article, he hoped it had "at last thrown all the dogs off my track" (December 5) [all quoted in F. Seward, supra note 1, pp. 478-80].

6. Seward December 2, 1860, letter to Weed ("If we can keep peace and quiet until the decree of S.C. is pronounced the temper will be favorable on both sides to conciliation.") (quoted in F. Seward, supra note 1, pp. 479-80) (see also Seward's December 7 letter to his wife (id. p. 480)). See also Seward December 11, 1860, letter to Hamilton Fish (Fish Papers, Library of Congress) (the Fire-Eaters rhetoric will show "the Border States that they are to be ruined by the licentiousness of the Gulf States if they go with them"); Stahr, supra note 3, p. 212; Crofts, supra note 4, pp. 219-20.

7. *A Compilation of the Messages and Papers of the Presidents, 1789-1897,* Volume 5, p. 626 (James D. Richardson ed.) (U.S. Government Printing Office 1896-1899). Buchanan also asked Northerners to repeal the various states' personal liberty laws, adopt a

constitutional amendment protecting slavery in the territories, and further advocated for the acquisition of Cuba (thus adding a large new slave state into the Union). See James McPherson, *Battle Cry of Freedom: The Civil War Era*, pp. 196-97 (Oxford University Press 1988).

8. Burlingame, supra note 2, Volume I, p. 707.

9. Seward December 5, 1860, letter to F. Seward (quoted in F. Seward, supra note 1, p. 480). When Seward later made this quip public, New York lawyer (and famed diarist) George Templeton Strong wrote that he did not believe "Bill Seward ever said anything so clever," *The Diary of George Templeton Strong*, Volume 3, p. 71 (eds. Allan Nevins & Milton Thomas) (Macmillan 1952).

10. According to Walter Stahr, there are at least three versions of the Hamlin-Seward conversation on December 12, 1860. Stahr, supra note 3, p. 597 n.11.

11. Abraham Lincoln December 8, 1860, letters to Seward (*The Collected Works of Abraham Lincoln*, Volume 4, pp. 148-49 (Roy Basler ed.) (Rutgers University Press 1953-55)). Michael Burlingame details the back-channel efforts of some of Seward's political foes to deep-six his appointment. Burlingame, supra note 2, Volume I, p. 721; see also Harold Holzer, *Lincoln President-Elect: Abraham Lincoln and the Great Secession Winter 1860-1861*, pp. 142-43 (Simon & Schuster 2008). Lincoln was undeterred: not only did he think Seward the preeminently qualified man for the position, as he told Edward Bates (soon to be Attorney General), if Seward refused his offer "that would excite bad feelings, and lead to a dangerous if not fatal rupture of the party." Burlingame, supra note 2, Volume I, p. 728.

12. C. Evan Stewart, "Diplomat of the Civil War," *New York Archives* (Summer 2011); Burlingame, supra note 2, Volume I, pp. 721-22.

13. On December 13, 1860, Seward wrote an initial letter responding to Lincoln's offer. Seward December 13, 1860, letter to Lincoln (Lincoln Papers, Library of Congress). Seward's letter three days earlier is also in the Lincoln Papers (and in F. Seward, supra note 1, p. 482).

14. Van Deusen, supra note 3, p. 240; Stahr, supra note 3, p. 215.

15. *Albany Evening Journal* (December 17, 1860) (Of course, this latter point essentially embraced the concept of Douglas's Popular Sovereignty, to which Lincoln had already made clear he could never agree. See supra Chapter IV, note 5.).

16. *Autobiography of Thurlow Weed*, pp. 603-04 (Harriet Weed ed.) (Houghton Mifflin 1883); David Potter, *Lincoln and His Party in the Secession Crisis*, p. 167 (Louisiana State University Press 1995).

17. Burlingame, supra note 2, Volume I, p. 712; Holzer, supra note 11, pp. 164-65; Potter, supra note 16, pp. 167-68. Lincoln also separately sent the three resolutions to Illinois Senator Lyman Trumbull. Lincoln December 21, 1860, letter to Trumbull (Basler, supra note 11, Volume 4, p. 158) ("I think it would be best for Mr. Seward to introduce them & Mr. Weed will let him know that I think so."). Lincoln's focus on the Fugitive Slave Act was not necessarily a misread of many of the Southern grievances. See Burlingame, supra note 2, Volume I, pp. 693-94. In fact, South Carolina's December 24, 1860, secession order justifying its action cites as the primary reason the North's flagrant non-enforcement of the Fugitive Slave Act. See also *Southern Pamphlets on Secession, November 1860-April 1861* (Jon Wakelyn ed.) (University of North Carolina Press 1996). Those

oft-repeated sentiments undoubtedly motivated Lincoln's focus on this issue. See also Chapter IV, note 5.

18. The most fulsome account of this meeting can be found in Holzer's *Lincoln President-Elect*, supra note 11, pp. 165-70; see also Weed ed., *Autobiography*, supra note 16, pp. 602-14; Thurlow W. Barnes, *Memoir of Thurlow Weed*, pp. 291-95 (Houghton Mifflin 1884); Crofts, supra note 4, pp. 221-22, 418 n.16; Stahr, supra note 3, pp. 216-17; Van Deusen, supra note 3, p. 240; Burlingame, supra note 2, Volume I, pp. 721-24.

19. The other men were Congressman Henry Winter Davis of Maryland (David B. Davis's cousin) and two former Congressmen: John Bolts of Virginia and Balie Peyton of Tennessee.

20. Lincoln, in fact, had just written to Gilmer, replying to an inquiry to "clarify" his views. Lincoln December 15, 1860 letter to Gilmer (Basler, supra note 11, Volume 4, pp. 151-52) (any further explanations "would make me appear as if I repented for the crime of having been elected, and was anxious to apologize and beg forgiveness."). Daniel Crofts provides an excellent, detailed account of Gilmer's political career (and potential use to a Lincoln administration) in *Reluctant Confederates*, supra note 4, pp. 24-26, 222-23. See also Daniel Crofts, "A Reluctant Unionist: John A. Gilmer and Lincoln's Cabinet," *Civil War History* (September 1978).

21. Blair would become the Postmaster General in 1861.

22. Bates would become the Attorney General in 1861.

23. While Lincoln and Weed liked each other and respected each's political sagacity, Weed came away from this meeting discouraged—to the point he counseled Seward on the wisdom of joining the cabinet. Weed December 25, 1860, letter to Seward (Seward Papers, University of Rochester); Van Deusen, supra note 3, p. 241; Burlingame, supra note 2, Volume I, p. 723.

24. *Congressional Globe*, p. 117 (Dec. 4, 1860); with respect to the House Committee see also Chapter IV, note 5.

25. See McPherson, supra note 7, pp. 198-99.

26. Potter, supra note 16, pp. 169-70; Stahr, supra note 3, p. 216.

27. *New York Times* (December 24, 1960); F. Seward, supra note 1, p. 483; Stahr, supra note 3, p. 217; Van Deusen, supra note 3, pp. 241-42.

28. Seward December 24, 1860, letter to F. Seward (F. Seward, supra note 1, p. 483).

29. As Lincoln explained to Pennsylvania Congressman James Hale, who was in favor of the Crittenden Compromise: "[I]f we surrender, it is the end of us, and of the government.... A year will not pass, till we have to take Cuba as a condition upon which they will stay in the Union." Lincoln January 11, 1861, letter to Hale (Basler, supra note 11, Volume 4, p. 172). For Stephen Douglas's rationale for supporting the Crittenden Compromise, see *The Letters of Stephen A. Douglas*, pp. 504-06 (Robert Johannsen ed.) (University of Illinois Press 1961) ("Nothing will do any good which does not take the slavery question out of Congress forever.").

30. Stahr, supra note 3, p. 218; Van Deusen, supra note 3, p. 243; Burlingame, supra note 2, Volume I, p. 746 (the Committee also rejected Douglas's proposal to bar blacks from voting or holding office; later, Douglas also proposed that free blacks be colonized to Africa or South America at federal expense). For an analysis of the Southern Committee members' openness to "Crittenden's blueprint or something similar," see "The Critical Signpost on the Journey Toward Secession" in Michael Cooper's *Approaching Civil War and Southern History*, pp. 125-38 (Louisiana State University Press 2019).

31. Seward December 26, 1860, letter to Lincoln (F. Seward, supra note 1, pp. 484-85); Stahr, supra note 3, pp. 218-19.

32. Each of these December 28 letters can be found at F. Seward, supra note 1, pp. 486-87. The day before Seward had met with Charles Francis Adams and discussed Lincoln's offer and his misgivings; Adams strongly urged Seward to accept the post "in this moment of great difficulty and danger." Stahr, supra note 3, p. 219; Van Deusen, supra note 3, p. 241. Seward, in explaining his decision to his wife, wrote: "I will try to save freedom and my country." Seward December 28, 1860, letter to F. Seward (F. Seward, supra note 1, p. 487).

33. Stahr, supra note 3, p. 220. The next day Seward wrote both Weed and Lincoln about how dangerous the Fort Sumter issue had become, going so far as to warn that "[a] plot is forming to seize the capitol on or before the 4th of March." Both letters of December 29 can be found at F. Seward, supra note 1, pp. 487-88; see also Stahr, supra note 3, p. 221.

This information came via a back-channel from President Buchanan's new Attorney General, Edward Stanton. Stahr, supra note 3, pp. 221-22; Van Deusen, supra note 1, p. 244; John M. Taylor, *William Henry Seward: Lincoln's Right Hand*, p. 131 (HarperCollins 1991). Lincoln, who would bring Stanton into his cabinet as Secretary of War in 1862, had gotten off to a rocky start with the sometimes gruff Staton on a legal case a few years before the 1860 election. Burlingame, supra note 2, Volume I, pp. 339-40 (Stanton had dismissed Lincoln's attempts to be helpful as co-counsel, referring to him as a "giraffe" and a "long-armed baboon"). Conversely, Stanton's work with Seward on some patent litigation had led to a personal friendship between the two men. Even historians not friendly to Seward have given him high marks on his personal charm and social skills with friend and foe alike. See David Potter, *Lincoln and His Party in the Secession Crisis*, p. 25 (Louisiana State University Press 1995 (originally Yale University Press 1942)); see also Stahr, supra note 3, p. 5; Van Deusen, supra note 1, pp. 255-61; Lawrence Denton, *William Henry Seward and the Secession Crisis*, pp. 58-59 (McFarland & Company 2009); Taylor, supra this note, pp. 90-91; Daniel Crofts, "Secession Winter: William Henry Seward and the Decision for War," *New York History* 230 (1984) and *Reluctant Confederates*, supra note 4, p. 235; Henry Adams, *The Education of Henry Adams*, p. 104 (Houghton Mifflin 1918). Indeed, notwithstanding that they were bitter rivals for political supremacy, Seward and Chase maintained a cordial social relationship. Walter Stahr, *Salmon Chase: Lincoln's Vital Rival*, p. 423 (Simon & Schuster 2021).

34. Van Deusen, supra note 3, pp. 243-44; Burlingame, supra note 2, Volume I, pp. 246-67; Daniel Crofts, supra note 33, at 241.

35. Russell McClintock, *Lincoln and the Decision for War*, p. 295 (University of North Carolina Press 2008); Burlingame, supra note 2, Volume I, pp. 715, 747; Denton, supra note 33, p. 71.

36. Burlingame, supra note 2, Volume I, p. 747. For the complicated legislative (and political) histories of these two compromise plans, see Crofts, *Reluctant Confederates*, supra note 4, pp. 200-14, 232-35, 241-42.

Chapter VI

January 1861—The "Premier" Speaks

As the New Year began things looked ominous. On January 9, 1861, not only did Mississippi follow South Carolina out of the Union, but a federal ship trying to re-supply Fort Sumter was fired upon and turned back as it tried to enter Charleston Harbor. Then, on January 10 and 11, first Florida and next Alabama seceded. During this same period the Virginia legislature was called into special session to consider secession.

With that backdrop, Seward intensified his multi-front initiatives to encourage Republicans on the Committee of Thirty-Three (led by Charles Francis Adams) to find common ground with Border State Unionists, while he continued his efforts to strengthen the latter group's political hand. Even historians not disposed to view Seward favorably have acknowledged that Seward "[d]ominat[ed] Congress" in his efforts to save the Union during this time period.[1]

One part of Seward's arsenal was to reach out to his wide group of political friends and foes and (choosing his words carefully) appear to be on as many sides of intractable issues as possible. Thus, for example, to James Barbour of Virginia, who told him that "nothing less than the Crittenden compromise" would keep his state in the fold, Seward replied: "I am of your opinion that nothing short of that will allay the excitement, and therefore I will favor it *substantially*."[2]

But behind his slight-of-hand political tactics lay the broad structures of Seward's "plan"—it consisted of three prongs:

- conciliate the Border State Unionists by coming up with some sort of compromise on territorial expansion (e.g., the New Mexico Plan, the Border State Plan)
- use Lincoln's three directives (hand delivered to Thurlow Weed) to strengthen Republican willingness to find some common ground with the Border State Unionists (notwithstanding Lincoln's "private" no

compromise directives to various Republican lawmakers in Washington)[3]

- change the choice/focus from slavery or freedom to Union or dis-Union and thereby use every means possible to gain time to arouse latent (but growing) Union sentiment in the Border States (and, conversely, prevent them from precipitously following the rash secession actions of the Cotton States.[4]

And Seward did not just share the elements of his plan with his friend and ally Charles Francis Adams. A few weeks later Lord Richard Lyons, the British minister to the United States, reported back to the Home Office:

> Mr. Seward's real view of the state of the country appears to be, that if bloodshed can be avoided until the new Government is installed, the seceding States will in no long time return to the Confederation. He has unbounded confidence in his own skill in managing the American people.... He thinks that in a few months the evils and hardships produced by Secession will become intolerably grievous to the

> Southern States; that they will be completely reassured as to the intentions of the Administration; and that the conservative element which is now kept under the surface by violent pressure of the Secessionists, will emerge with irresistible force. From all these causes he confidently expects that when elections . . . are held in the Southern States in November next, the Union Parties will have a clear majority, and will bring the Seceding States back into the Confederation.[5]

To help in the implementation of Seward's plan, came the January 9 announcement in Thurlow Weed's paper (the *Albany Evening Journal*) of what had been long rumored: Lincoln had chosen Seward to serve as Secretary of State in the new administration. Weed wrote that Seward would be the "premier" to Lincoln's president, and that together they would "discharge their duties, amid all the difficulties that surround them, so as to preserve the blessing of Union, and to deserve and receive the homage of their countrymen."[6] With news of his appointment now broadly disseminated, Seward announced that he would address the Senate on January 12 (a Saturday).

Believing Seward would be speaking for the new administration, Horace Greeley's *New York Tribune* wrote that "the next premier['s] ... words will be scrutinized with much precision."[7] Thus, when Seward rose to speak at one p.m. on the January 12, approximately 2,000 people were jammed into the Senate (including virtually the entire Senate (and their wives), Senators from states that had seceded (e.g., Jefferson Davis), and most of Buchanan's cabinet).[8]

The Speech (And Its Aftermath)

At the outset, Seward invoked the sanctity of the Union (it "is not more the body than liberty is the soul of the nation"), cited the multiple benefits that had accrued to all the states since the founding of the country, and predicted calamities if the Union were dissolved.[9] And he enumerated a list of what "would *not* save [the Union]"—included in that list: "a continuation of the debate over slavery in the Territories," "proving that secession is illegal," discussing the right of the Federal Government "to coerce seceding States," and "Congressional compromise." Then he turned to the concessions he would make to prevent "perpetual civil war" (the direct consequence of the dissolution of the Union)[10]—there were five:

1. all state laws in conflict with the Constitution (e.g., the personal liberty laws) would be repealed;
2. a constitutional amendment would be enacted to ensure that slavery could not be interfered with "in any state";
3. Kansas should be admitted as a free state, with the remaining Western territory being divided into two additional states (implying New Mexico would come in as a slave state); alternatively, a constitutional convention should be held in a few years (after passions had cooled down) to consider the status of the Western territory and any related issues;
4. to deter another incident like John Brown's invasion of Virginia to foment a slave insurrection, Congress should enact a law to "prevent mutual invasions of states by citizens of other states";
5. there should be two separate railroads constructed to reach the Pacific—a Northern one and a Southern one.[11]

Citing the "example of the noble Senator from Tennessee" (Andrew Johnson—later to become Lincoln's vice president, then successor), Seward "avow[ed his] adherence to the Union in its integrity and with all its parts":

> I know we are in the midst of alarms and somewhat exposed to accidents. We already have disorder, and violence has begun. I know not to what extent it may go. Still my faith in the Constitution and in the Union abides. Whatever dangers there shall be, there will be the determination to meet them. Whatever sacrifices, private or public, shall be needful for the Union, they will be made. I feel sure that the hour has not come for this great nation to fail.

Reactions to the speech were widely different: Radical Republicans and abolitionists denounced it (including Seward's own wife!)[12]; and the secessionist wing of the Democrats did too.[13] But neither group was the audience to which Seward was appealing. Importantly, as the *New York Times* reported, leading border states representatives were "highly pleased" by the speech and "the people ... who represent the conservative spirit of the South [] are in fine spirits."[14] And as Lincoln wrote to Seward, the speech "is well received here [in Springfield], and, I think, is doing good all over the country."[15]

Lincoln was right, because a few days later the Virginia legislature rejected convening a secession convention[16]; instead, a process was established to have a vote regarding a convention on February 4, with the process skewed against secession. The legislature also called for a "Peace Convention" consisting of all states to take place in Washington starting in the first week of February.[17] Henry Adams (Congressman Adams's youngest son) would later credit Seward's "hidden-hand" behind the idea of a "Peace Convention"[18]; whether true or not, the process allowed Seward to continue his efforts to strengthen Union sentiment in the Upper South.[19]

But Lincoln was still resisting any compromise on the extension of slavery, and Seward recognized that without the president-elect indicating some flexibility there would likely be no way to bolster sufficient Union support in the Upper South. Seward's first attempt to bend Lincoln's intransigence was to send Illinois Congressman William Kellogg (a member of the Committee of Thirty-Three) to Springfield to visit Lincoln in late January. Although Lincoln reiterated his openness to a Constitutional convention, he said he would not compromise on slavery's expansion.[20] Somewhat incongruously, Kellogg came back to Washington ("full of compromise"), reporting to his Border State colleagues that "something must and will be done soon" on which they could "stand."[21] And while it looked like a modified Border State plan might cobble together enough votes, confusion as to where Lincoln really stood proved to be an insurmountable obstacle.[22] As such, on January 27 Seward wrote to Lincoln that

> [t]he appeals from the Union men in the Border states for something of concession or compromise are very painful since they say that without it those states must go with the tide, and your administration must begin with the free states, meeting all the Southern states in a hostile confederacy.... It is almost in vain that I tell them to wait, let us have a truce on slavery, put our issue on Disunion and seek remedies for ultimate grief in a constitutional question.... [E]very thought that we think ought to be conciliatory, forebearing and patient, and so open the way for the rising of a Union Party in the seceding states which will bring them back into the Union.[23]

Notes

1. Michael Burlingame, *Abraham Lincoln: A Life*, Volume I, pp. 707, 745-46 (Johns Hopkins University Press 2009); David

Potter, *Lincoln and His Party in the Secession Crisis*, pp. 240-44 (Louisiana State University Press 1995 (originally Yale University Press 1942)); Walter Stahr, *Seward: Lincoln's Indispensable Man*, pp. 242-43 (Simon & Schuster 2012); Glyndon Van Deusen, *William Henry Seward* (Oxford University Press 1967); see also Daniel Crofts's 1995 Introduction to Potter's book (pp. xix-xxii). Seward, in fact, wrote his wife that he had "assumed a sort of dictatorship for defense.... My hope, rather my confidence, is unabated." (Frederick W. Seward, *Seward at Washington: 1846-61*, pp. 490-91 (Derby and Miller 1891)). The Adams family agreed, viewing Seward as the "virtual ruler of this country" during the Secession Winter. Henry Adams January 17, 1861, letter to Charles Francis Adams Jr. (*Letters of Henry Adams*, Volume I, p. 223 (J.C. Levenson ed.) (Harvard University Press 1982-1988)); see also Burlingame, supra this note, Volume I, p. 745.

2. Frederick Bancroft, *The Life of William H. Seward*, Volume 2, p. 320 (Harper & Row 1900). For other examples of Seward's political feints and dekes—attempting to delay (at a minimum) precipitous actions—see Van Deusen, supra note 1, pp. 247-48; Daniel Crofts, "Secession Winter: William Henry Seward and the Decision of War," *New York History* 240 (July 1984). Not surprisingly some of the never-compromise Republicans were not enchanted by Seward's political slight-of-hands. See Burlingame, supra note 1, Volume I, pp. 752-53; Charles Sumner February 6, 1861, letter to J. Andrew, *The Selected Letters of Charles Sumner*, Volume 2, pp. 55-56 (Beverly Palmer ed.) (Northeastern University Press 1990) (with respect to the New Mexico plan, "*Seward will not vote for it*. He will use it as a lure; *but not vote for it*."). Southern Fire-Eaters also were unhappy with Seward's efforts, fearing they might well work. Lawrence Denton, *William Henry Seward and the Secession Crisis*, pp. 75-76 (McFarland & Company 2009).

3. As Lincoln's foremost biographer has noted: "in objecting to all compromise measures, Lincoln was out of step with the members of his party in Congress who were better informed about affairs in the South and more alarmed as threats of secession became reality." David Donald, *Lincoln*, p. 269 (Simon & Schuster 1996). See also James Rhodes, *History of the United States from 1850 to 1877*, Volume 3, p. 261 (Macmillan 1910) (if the Crittenden Proposal "had been submitted to the people [in January 1861] it would have carried the Northern States by a great majority; ... it would have obtained the vote of almost every man in the border States; and ... it would have received the preponderating voice of all the Cotton States but South Carolina.").

4. Van Deusen, supra note 1, pp. 242-43; Denton, supra note 2, p. 69; John M. Taylor, *William Henry Seward: Lincoln's Right Hand*, p. 130 (HarperCollins 1991).

5. Richard Lyons February 4, 1861, letter to John Russell (*The American Civil War Through British Eyes*, Volume I, p. 28 (James Barnes & Patricia Barnes eds.) (Kent State University Press 2003-05); Stahr, supra note 1, pp. 232-33; Taylor, supra note 4, p. 133; Burlingame, supra note 1, Volume I, p. 746. Lyons ended his report, observing that Seward "hopes to place himself at the head of a strong Union party, having extensive ramifications both in the North and in the South, and to make Union or Disunion not Freedom or Slavery the watchword of political parties," adding that "in all this" Seward assumes "Lincoln will leave the whole management of affairs to him." Seward delivered a similar message to Russian Minister Baron Edouard de Stoecki. Van Deusen, supra note 1, p. 247. And he also (foreshadowing his famous/infamous April 1, 1861, memorandum ("Some Thoughts for the President's Consideration")) (see infra Chapter IX) talked to many foreign ministers in Washington about

stirring up trouble with foreign nations as "the best means of re-establishing internal peace." Stahr, supra note 1, p. 231; Van Deusen, supra note 1, pp. 247-48.

6. *Albany Evening Journal* (January 9-11, 1861); Stahr, supra note 1, p. 223. (See also the *New York Times* (January 9-11, 1861). Salmon Chase, Seward's political archnemesis in the first term of Lincoln's administration, congratulated Seward on this appointment. Chase January 10, 1861, letter to Seward (Seward Papers, University of Rochester) ("the post is yours by right and you will honor the post. My best wishes go with you.") On that same day Chase woke to a political ally: "[Lincoln] could not do otherwise than offer the first position in his Administration to Mr. Seward …, Mr. Seward by his own abilities, by the voice of New York, by the consent of the press and by the sentiment of a great majority of the Republicans has been made our foremost man and Mr. Lincoln might well feel himself constrained to tender him the position he has accepted." Chase January 10, 1861, letter to J.S. Pike, *The Salmon P. Chase Papers,* Volume 3, pp. 46-48 (John Niven ed.) (Kent State University Press 1996). Lincoln would subsequently write Seward that, with the public announcement, "I am happy to find scarcely any objection to it." Lincoln January 11, 1861, letter to Seward (F. Seward, supra note 1, p. 493).

7. *New York Tribune* (January 11, 1861); see also *Washington Evening Star* (January 11-12, 1861) (Seward would deliver "the most momentous" speech "ever delivered before that body" and "the Union may yet escape destruction.").

8. Van Deusen, supra note 1, p. 244; Stahr, supra note 1, p. 223.

9. *Congressional Globe,* pp. 341-44. There are innumerable (and often quite differing) accounts of Seward's Senate speech (and

reactions thereto). See F. Seward, supra note 1, pp. 493-95; Potter, supra note 1, pp. 285-88; Daniel Crofts, *Reluctant Confederates: Upper South Unionists in the Secession Crisis*, pp. 236-37 (University of North Carolina Press 1987); Stahr, supra note 1, pp. 223-26; Van Deusen, supra note 1, pp. 244-46; Taylor, supra note 4, pp. 134-35; Denton, supra note 2, pp. 79-80; Harold Holzer, *Lincoln President-Elect: Abraham Lincoln and the Great Secession Winter 1860-1861*, pp. 214-15 (Simon & Schuster 2008); Burlingame, supra note 1, Volume I, pp. 747-48. For example, Frederick Seward and Stahr both reported that Senator John Crittenden was moved to tears by Seward's eloquence; Burlingame, on the other hand, reported that Crittenden's reaction to Seward's words was one of despair because "all hope seem to have fled."

10. Anticipating that an enumeration of unilateral concessions would be perceived by many (especially no-compromise Republicans—i.e., Sumner, Chase, etc.) as a big pill to swallow, Seward said that many of his proposals did not arise from his own "cherished convictions," offering this rationale:

> I learned from Jefferson that, in political affairs, we cannot always do what seems to us absolutely best.... We must be content to lead when we can, and to follow when we cannot lead; and if we cannot ... do for our country all the good we could wish, we must be satisfied with doing for her all the good we can.

Bancroft, supra note 2, Volume 2, p. 15; see also Taylor, supra note 4, p. 135.

As noted above, however (see supra note 3), Seward's conciliatory impulses were more in keeping with a large number of Republican lawmakers in Washington.

11. As noted earlier (see Chapter I, note 7), Seward believed that an even greater issue was fulfilling America's destiny as a commercial (and otherwise) empire, spanning the continent and reaching across the Pacific Ocean.

12. Not surprisingly, Michael Burlingame assembled a litany of Radical Republican reactions (including that of Thaddeus Stevens). Burlingame, supra note 1, Volume I, pp. 747-48. Senator Charles Sumner (a leading Radical Republican) wrote to one correspondent: "Many republicans regretted that [Seward] should deem it his duty to make *offers* or *concessions* of any kind. It seems to me that the North has one duty; quietly, calmly, but firmly to stand by its principles. The crisis will soon pass." To another he wrote: "I deplore S[eward]'s speech. He read it to me 4 days before its delivery & I protested with all the earnestness of my soul & all the strength of language I could command against his propositions—*against any propositions*. I fear it will demoralize the Northern sentiments." Charles Sumner January 14, 1861, letter to D. Dix and January 17, 1861, letter to J. Jay, *The Selected Letters of Charles Sumner*, supra note 2, Volume 2, pp. 41-43; see also Stahr, p. 225.

Francis Seward, who was a true abolitionist (see Dorothy Wickenden, "Civil Wars," *The New Yorker* 16-25 (January 25, 2021)), rebuked her husband, telling him he was "in danger of taking the path which led Daniel Webster to an unhonored grave ten years ago [when he supported the Compromise of 1850, which included the Fugitive Slave Act]. Compromises based on the idea that the preservation of the Union is more important than the liberty of 4,000,000 human beings cannot be right. The alteration of the Constitution to perpetuate slavery—the enforcement of a law to recapture a poor, suffering fugitive—giving half of the Territories of a free country to the course of slavery—these compromises cannot be approved by

God or supported by good men." F. Seward January 19, 1861, letter to Seward (Seward Papers, University of Rochester).

In letters back to his wife, Seward wrote he was

> not surprised that [she did] not like the "concessions" in my speech. You will soon enough come to see that they are not compromises, but explanations to disarm the enemies of Truth, Freedom, and Union, of their most effective weapons.
>
> * * *
>
> My own party trusts me, but not without reservations. All the other parties, North and South, cast themselves upon me.
>
> * * *
>
> I must gain time for the new Administration to organize and for the frenzy of passion to subside. I am doing this without making any compromise whatever, by forbearance, conciliation, magnanimity.

Seward January 18 and 23, 1861, letters to F Seward (F. Seward, supra note 1, pp. 496-97).

Mrs. Seward's citation to Daniel Webster merits further comment. When Webster had made his famous speech in 1850, John Greenleaf Whittier (a poet) had denounced him: "So fallen! So lost! The light withdrawn which once he wore!" But Whittier's response to Seward's 1861 speech was very different. In the *New York Evening Post* (January 25, 1861), he published this poem:

> To William H. Seward.
> Statesman. I thank thee!—and, if yet dissent
> Mingles, reluctant, with my larger content.

I cannot censure what was nobly meant,
But, while constrained to hold even Union less
Than Liberty and Truth and Righteous news,
I thank thee in the sweet and holy name
Of Peace, for wise calm words that put to shame
Passion and party. Courage may be shown
Not in defiance of the wrong alone;
He may be bravest who, unweaponed, bears
The olive branch, and strong in justice, spares
The rash wrong-doer, giving widest scope
To Christian charity and generous hope.
If, without damage to the sacred cause
Of Freedom and the safeguard of its laws—
If, without yielding that for which alone
We prize the Union, thou canst save it now
From a baptism of blood, upon thy brow
A wreath whose flowers no earthly soul has known,
Woven of the beatitudes, shall rest;
And the peacemaker be forever blest.

Crofts, supra note 2, pp. 243-44. According to Henry Adams, the only time during this entire period Seward showed real emotion was when "he opened the envelope and read the sonnet which the poet Whittier sent to him from Amesbury." Henry Adams, "The Great Secession Winter of 1860-61," *Proceedings of the Massachusetts Historical Society*, p. 685 (1910).

13. For a sampling of secessionist reactions see Crofts, supra note 2, pp. 236-37.

14. *New York Times* (January 16, 1861).

15. Lincoln January 19, 1861, letter to Seward (Roy Basler (ed.), *The Collected Works of Abraham Lincoln*, Volume 4, p. 176 (Rutgers University Press 1953-55)). Some historians (based on hearsay) believe Lincoln was "not overpleased with Seward's speech" (with Lincoln also telling Carl Schurz that "Seward made all his speeches without consulting him"). Holzer, supra note 9, pp. 214-15; Burlingame, supra note 1, Volume I, pp. 748, 746. If true, then Honest Abe (in Holzer's words) was "perhaps [engaged in] a somewhat disingenuous attempt to have it both ways."

The actual contemporaneous record does not appear to support Holzer's conclusion(s) vis-à-vis Lincoln attempting to have it both ways. A Springfield, Illinois, paper (which published Lincoln's views) praised Seward's speech, and supported the call for a Constitutional convention, noting that the process for establishing such a convention "will take *time*, and time is all that is necessary to cure the secession fever." *Illinois State Journal* (February 6, 1861). And Lincoln's aide, John Hay, wrote in another newspaper: "I have reason to believe [Lincoln] coincides with Gov. Seward in favoring a convention of the people to suggest amendment to the Constitution," *Missouri Democrat* (January 21, 1861). See also Burlingame, supra note 1, Volume I, p. 748.

16. Crofts, supra note 9, pp. 137-38.

17. The leading studies of the Peace Conference are Mark Tooley's *The Peace That Almost Was: The Forgotten Story of the 1861 Peace Conference and the Final Attempt to Avert the Civil War* (Nelson Books 2015) and Robert Gunderson's *Old Gentlemen's Convention* (University of Wisconsin Press 1961). See also David Bahr, "The Talking Game: One Last Effort to Avoid Civil War," *The Weekly Standard* (December 7, 2015).

18. Potter, supra note 1, pp. 307-08; Van Deusen, supra note 1, p. 248; Denton, supra note 2, p. 207; James McPherson also gives credit to Seward's "hidden-hand" (see James McPherson, *Battle Cry of Freedom: The Civil War Era*, p. 201 (Oxford University Press 1988)); see also Crofts, supra note 2, p. 245; Adams, supra note 12, p. 24; Patrick Sowle, "The Conciliatory Republicans During the Winter of Secession," p. 276 (Ph.D. Dissertation) (Duke University 1963). Stahr nonetheless calls the evidence of Seward's hidden-hand "rather thin" (supra note 1, p. 227).

This linkage is undoubtedly due to the fact that the key Virginia Unionists driving this result—Whig George Summers and Democrat James Barbour—were in constant contact with Seward during the Secession Winter. See Crofts, supra note 9, pp. 138, 264, 267-68, 270, 275-76, 289, 308.

19. Seward's frenetic efforts at this moment are well-documented in Crofts's *Reluctant Confederates*, supra note 9, pp. 205-06. At a large dinner party hosted by Stephen Douglas on January 24 Seward toasted: "Away with all parties, all platforms of previous committals, and whatever else will stand in the way of the restoration of the American Union!" Senator Crittenden's response was so emphatic that his class "shivered to fragments." Taylor, supra note 4, p. 134; Denton, supra note 2, p. 82.

20. Burlingame, supra note 1, Volume I, p. 748; Holzer, supra note 9, pp. 240-41.

21. Crofts, supra note 9, pp. 207, 242; Denton, supra note 2, pp. 82-84. It is possible that Kellogg's optimism was based on the flexibility regarding New Mexico that Lincoln evidenced in his February 1 letter to Seward (see infra Chapter VII notes 1-3 and text); but I have found no record of Lincoln giving Kellogg any such

indication. See Paul Angle (ed.), "The Recollections of William Pitt Kellogg," *The Abraham Lincoln Quarterly* (September 1945).

22. Crofts, supra note 9, pp. 207-14. No-compromise Republicans (e.g., Illinois Congressman E.B. Washburne) were always on the lookout for "compromise that is supposed to be hatching by the Weed-Seward dynasty ... [designed] to obtain your acquiescence in the scheme to sell out and degrade the republicans." Washburne January 7, 1861, letter to Lincoln (*The Lincoln Papers,* Volume 2, p. 390 (David Mearns ed.) (Doubleday 1948)); see also Holzer, supra note 9, pp. 215-16; Crofts, supra note 9, p. 242; Stahr, supra note 1, p. 235 (Chase's efforts to block Seward's appointment).

23. Seward January 27, 1861, letter to Lincoln (Lincoln Papers, Library of Congress); see Stahr, supra note 1, pp. 230-31; Denton, supra note 2, pp. 86-87.

Chapter VII

February 1861—A Very Busy Month

Seward's plea of January 27 seemed to touch a chord. In his February 1 response, Lincoln wrote to Seward, reiterating his (still private) opposition to a compromise on slavery's expansion, but adding:

> As to fugitive slaves, District of Columbia, slave trade among slave states, and whatever springs of necessity from the fact that the institution is amongst us, I care but little.... *Nor do I care much about New Mexico, if further extension were hedged against.* (Emphasis added.)[1]

Upon receiving Lincoln's letter, Seward told Congressman Adams that Lincoln "approved his course."[2] But Seward did not see *any* compromise garnering enough support at that point and did not want to risk "making himself responsible for a rejected plan" (according to Lord Richard Lyons, Britain's Ambassador to the United States); indeed, as Seward told a New York group espousing a variation of the Crittenden Compromise, if he backed a losing plan he would be finished politically and "would have to go back to Auburn and amuse myself with writing history the rest of my life."[3] Instead, with the Peace Convention just

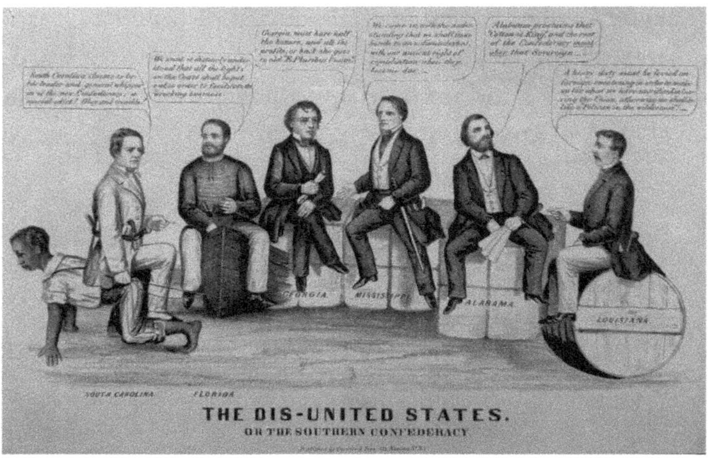

The Dis-United States or the Southern Confederacy
(1861 drawing by Louis Maurer; published by Courier & Ives)
(author's collection)

getting underway in Washington,[4] Seward continued his back-channel efforts to strengthen Union sentiment in the Upper South.

And those efforts seemed to be moving the needle. At the same time that representatives of the seven seceded states were meeting in Montgomery, Alabama, to hammer out the details of a Confederate government (February 4), the Peace Conference (led by ex-President John Tyler) got underway in Washington.[5] Far more important than the Peace Conference, however, was the fact that Virginia voters were also at the polls to select delegates to a secession convention. By the next day it was clear that all of Seward's interactions with Virginia's leading Union men (especially James Barbour and George Summers) had in fact borne fruit. Of the 152 delegates elected, fewer than one-third favored secession. Virginia voters also endorsed a process whereby any secession decision by a convention would have to be subject to a statewide referendum (by a 103,236 to 46,386 margin).[6]

This news was exactly what Seward had planned and hoped for. As reported in the *New York Evening Post,* "Mr. Seward, with his characteristic hope and confidence, is particularly pleased with the result. He pronounces the Union safe, and that all the border states will follow the example of the Old Dominion."[7]

Of particular importance was the fact that the Virginia election had "annihilated all existing party organization" and suggested "a fundamental rearrangement of political forces in the state"—with the defining issue *not* expansion of slavery, but rather: "UNION or DISUNION."[8]

Just a few days later (on February 9) Tennessee voters delivered an even stronger pro-Union message. By a vote of 69,772 to 57,708, they rejected even holding a state convention to consider secession.[9] In the midst of all this good news, Henry Adams recorded:

> The ancient Seward is in high spirits and chuckles himself hoarse with his stories. He says it's all right. We shall keep the border states, and in three months or thereabouts, if we hold off, the Unionists and Disunionists will have their hands on each other's throats in the cotton states. The storm is weathered.[10]

But just as things looked most promising for Seward's pro-Union efforts, the tide turned. Lincoln, who had rejected Seward's December 28 suggestion that he come to Washington earlier than planned to gauge for himself the turbulent climate in the Capitol,[11] had now decided to change his public period of "masterly inactivity." On February 11, Lincoln left Springfield for a meandering railroad journey in route to Washington, across most of the Northern states that had elected him; he wanted to see the people and wanted them to see him.[12] Unfortunately, the trip, in many ways, was a debacle.

Lincoln's Railroad Speeches

On the first evening of the journey, the train stopped in Indianapolis, Indiana. Speaking extemporaneously from the balcony of his hotel, Lincoln launched into an exposition on the relationship of the states to the federal government, and that led to definitional explanations of the words "coerced" and "invasion." If the federal government "simply insists upon holding its own forts, or *retaking* those forts that belong to it [cheers],—or the enforcement of the laws of the United States in the collection of duties upon foreign importations [renewed cheers], ... would any of those things be coercion?"[13]

Days later, in Columbus, Ohio, Lincoln (again, speaking off the cuff) told the Ohio legislature:

> I have not maintained silence from any want of real anxiety. It is a good thing that there is no more anxiety, for there is *nothing going wrong*. It

> is a consulting circumstance that when we look out, there is *nothing that really hurts anybody*.[14]

From there the train moved on to Pittsburgh, Pennsylvania, where the president-elect told a large audience (standing in the rain) that "there is really no crisis except an *artificial* one."[15] After a lengthy visit in heavily Democratic New York City, which Lincoln survived without any major verbal gaffes,[16] the train moved on to New Jersey. Addressing the state senate in Trenton, Lincoln assured the legislators that no man desired peace more than he: "But it may be necessary to put the foot down firmly." And as he said those words (according to his aide, John Hay), Lincoln "lifted his foot lightly, and pressed it with a quick, but not violent gesture upon the floor." This brought "shouts and cheers and yells and shrieks," and it was minutes before Lincoln could continue.[17]

In Washington, D.C. (and beyond), Lincoln's impromptu remarks (which had been widely publicized) had a profound impact. Not only did they make it seem that Lincoln would make *no* conciliatory gestures to help Southern Unionists, they also undercut the notion that Seward's efforts of the past several months had been with Lincoln's blessing (thereby undercutting Seward's purported "Premier" role in the new administration).[18]

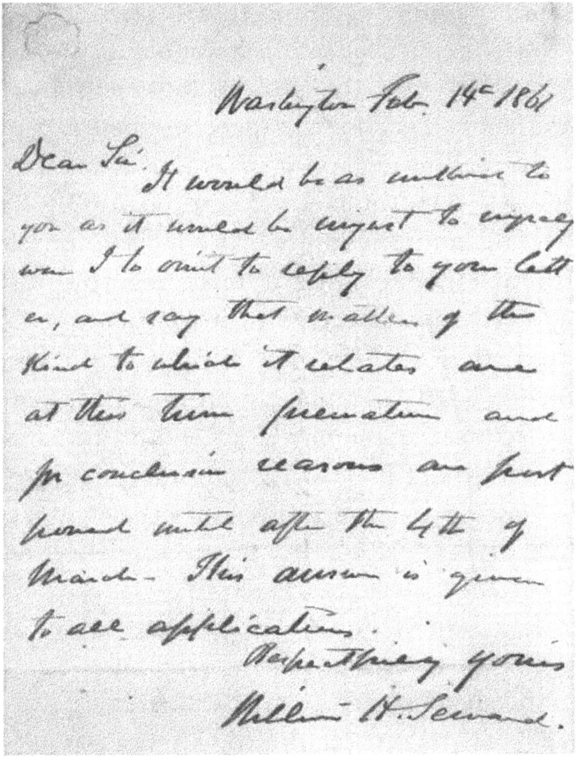

Washington Feb. 14th 1861

Dear Sir,

It would be as unkind to you as it would be unjust to myself were I to omit to reply to your letter, and say that matters of the kind to which it relates are at this time premature and for conclusive reasons are best housed until after the 4th of March. This answer is given to all applications.

Respectfully yours

William H. Seward.

Seward February 14, 1861, letter regarding the impending presidential inauguration
["It would be as unkind to you as it would be unjust to myself were I to omit to reply to your letter, and say that matters of the kind to which it relates are at this time premature and for conclusive reasons are best housed until after the 4th of March. This answer is given to all applications."]
(author's collection)

Charles Francis Adams told a friend that Lincoln's "speeches have fallen like a wet blanket here." And in his diary he wrote that "in this lottery we may have drawn a blank," because the speeches "betray a person unconscious of his own position as well as the nature of the contest around him. Good natured, kindly, honest, but frivolous and uncertain.... I confess I am gloomy about him. His beginning is most inauspicious." His son reported that Seward and his father were "more depressed" than at any prior time because Lincoln's speeches had left Virginia Unionists "in despair"—if Lincoln followed the policy he uttered in Indianapolis, they could "do nothing" to prevent Virginia from leaving the Union.[19] And on February 19 the Congressman told his family:

> [T]en days before, the whole game was in Seward's hands; but now it is surrendered again to the chapter of accidents. The difficulty was wholly owing to Lincoln's folly in not consulting both his official advisors, but saying whatever came into his head. Thus he was dividing the party deplorably—destroying the chance of union inaction. Seward's position had thus been made lamentable; for, with his strength exhausted he was surrounded by opponents,

> friends, and foes; and here now was Lincoln, without consultation or understanding with Seward, and with no apparent regard for the policy indicated by him, showing an ignorance as complete as lamentable of the position of public affairs, fomenting discussions and jealousies already too formidable.[20]

And it was not just Seward, the Adams family, and Border State Unionists laid low by Lincoln's railroad speeches, a broad swatch of the body politic thought them regrettable (and unhelpful to finding an acceptable *modus vivendi* to the crisis). For example, Edward Everett (former president of Harvard and the vice presidential candidate on the Constitutional Union Party ticket) opined: "He is evidently a person of very inferior cast of character, wholly unequal to the crisis." And even Lincoln admirers such as George Templeton Strong (New York lawyer and famed diarist) would "have been better pleased with [Lincoln] if he had held his tongue altogether."[21]

With Seward trying to react to these new obstacles and think of a way forward, yet another problem arose: credible reports came that an attempt would be made on Lincoln's life as his train passed through the City of Baltimore—a hotbed of secession fever.[22]

Avoiding Assassination

On February 21, General Winfield Scott (head of the U.S. Army) sent a note to Seward about the plot. Seward summoned his son, Frederick (who was in the Senate gallery), and told him:

> Find Mr. Lincoln, wherever he is. Let no one else know your errand. I have written him that I think he should change his arrangements, and pass through Baltimore at a different hour. I know it may occasion some embarrassment, and perhaps, some ill-natured talk. Nevertheless, I would strongly advise him to do it.[23]

Frederick Seward took a train to Philadelphia and, after being prescreened by Lincoln's son, Robert, he met with the president-elect at about 11 p.m. Because Lincoln had independently heard of other such threats, he and his advisors traveling with him (principally his friend and bodyguard, Colonel Ward Hill Lamon) decided he should act on Seward's instruction and not follow the well-published itinerary. Frederick Seward thereupon telegraphed his father a code word "previously agreed upon," which confirmed that Lincoln would follow Seward's advice. And so Lincoln (stooping over and described to the railroad conductor as an invalid) boarded the 10:50 p.m. sleeping car compartment of the train (together with Lamon and famed detective, Allen Pinkerton); the three men went unnoticed when the train reached Baltimore at 3:30 a.m. Ultimately, the train reached Washington at 6 a.m. on February 23.[24] It was met by Illinois Congressman E.B. Washburn, who accompanied the men "by hack" to the Willard Hotel.[25]

Lincoln in Washington

For the next few days Seward officiated as Lincoln's tour guide to official Washington (visiting the President, the Senate, the House, the Supreme Court), and attended church and broke bread with him. During these events Seward used all of his considerable one-on-one charm not only to convince the president-elect to evidence conciliation to the Border State Unionists but also to lobby for a more conciliatory Cabinet.[26]

Those latter efforts seemed for naught when Lincoln, upon polling Senate Republicans, decided to follow through with the appointment of Salmon Chase to be Secretary of the Treasury. Because of that nomination, John Gilmer—realizing that the no-compromise wing of the incoming administration was on the rise (and Seward's "dominance" would recede)—decided to refuse a cabinet position (which had the corollary of pulling Montgomery Blair—another no-compromiser—into the cabinet).[27] This double whammy was, in Henry Adams's words, "the death blow to the policy of Mr. Seward."[28]

Nonetheless, having been asked by Lincoln to comment on his draft Inaugural Address,[29] Seward on Sunday evening (February 24) sent a lengthy letter to Lincoln, along with a marked-up copy of the inaugural draft with some 50 suggested changes.[30] In his cover letter (and comments), Seward seemed to channel the remarks he had made to the "Wide Awakes" on the night of the election:[31]

> *My Dear Sir*—I have suggested many changes, of little importance, severally, but in their general effect, tending to sooth the public mind.
>
> Of course the concessions are, as they ought to be, if they are to be of avail, at the cost of the winning, the triumphant party. I do not fear their displeasure. They will be loyal, whatever is said. Not so the defeated, irritated, angered, frenzied party. I, my dear sir, have devoted myself singly to the study of the case—here, with advantage of access and free communication with all parties of all sections. I have a common responsibility and interest

with you, and I shall adhere to you faithfully in every case. You must, therefore, allow me to speak frankly and candidly. In this spirit I declare to you that my convictions that the *second* and *third* paragraphs, even if modified as I propose in my amendments, will give advantage to the Disunionists, that Virginia and Maryland will secede; and we shall have within ninety, perhaps within sixty days, be obliged to fight the South for this capital, with a divided North for our reliance; and we shall not have one loyal magistrate or ministerial office south of the Potomac.

In that case the dismemberment of the Republic would date from the inauguration of a Republican Administration. I, therefore, most respectfully counsel the omission of those paragraphs. I know the tenacity of party friends; and I honor and respect it. But I know also that they know nothing of the real peril of the crisis. It has not been their duty to study it, as it has been mine. Only the soothing words which I have spoken have saved us and carried us along thus far. Every loyal man, and indeed, every disloyal man in the South, will tell you thus.

Your case is quite like that of *Jefferson*. He brought the first Republican party into power against and over a party ready to resist and dismember the Government. Partisan as he was, he sank the partisan in the patriot, in his inaugural address; and propitiated his adversaries by declaring, "We are all Federalists; all Republicans." I could wish that you would think it wise to follow this example, in this crisis. Be sure that while your administrative conduct will be in harmony with Republican principles and policy, you cannot lose the Republican party by practicing, in your advent to office, the magnanimity of a victor.

Very faithfully your friend,

WILLIAM H. SEWARD

General Remarks

The argument is strong and conclusive, and ought not to be in any way abridged or modified.

But something besides, or in addition to argument is needful, to meet and remove *prejudice* and *passion* in the *South* and *fear* in the

> *East*. Some words of affection Some of calm and cheerful confidence.[32]

Seward's suggested changes covered six pages, and (as indicated by his cover letter) they were principally aimed at toning down the hard-line rhetoric aimed at the South. Besides advising Lincoln to delete the second and third paragraphs (referencing Lincoln's fidelity to the Republican Convention's platform) as too partisan, Seward advised deleting a scalding reference to the Supreme Court (author of the *Dred Scott* decision) ("the despotism of the few life officers"). And where Lincoln had labeled attacks on federal property as "treasonable," Seward suggested "revolutionary". With respect to Lincoln's language about the federal government's role vis-à-vis federal forts in the South (most particularly Fort Sumter), Seward recommended taking out "to reclaim the public property and places which have fallen," and suggested instead language whereby any enforcement of federal laws in the Southern states would be done with a view of "the circumstances actually existing, and a view and a hope of peaceful solutions of the national troubles and the restoration of fraternal sympathies and affection."[33] Most important was Seward's advice to drop Lincoln's ending—a "bellicose challenge" to the seceded states.[34]

Seward's cover letter and comments had been rewritten by his son (who had much more readable handwriting). But Seward hand wrote his proposed ending (with his own editing intact); it read as follows:

> I close. We are not we must not be aliens or enemies but fellow countrymen and brethren. Although passion has strained our bonds of affection too hardly they must not, I am sure they will not be broken. The mystic chords which proceeding from so many battle fields and so many patriot graves pass through all the hearts and in this broad continent of ours will yet again harmonize in their ancient music when breathed upon by the better guardian angel of the nation.[35]

What Lincoln would do with Seward's comments was not clear.[36] During the last week of February 1861, Lincoln's time was mainly focused on the messy business of locking down the various cabinet positions, while juggling the vicious infighting and jockeying for position that was taking place (and which always seems inevitable at the highest levels of government).[37] One other incident of significance (to this story) took up the president-elect's time: the conclusion of the Washington Peace Conference.

The End of the Peace Conference

After weeks of endless debates, arguments, and attempts at compromise, the Peace Conference ultimately endorsed a quasi-Border State plan on February 26 and referred it to Congress.[38] But with little appeal to Republicans (especially the president-elect), it stood no chance of Congressional approval. As such, it was rejected (with Seward (as explained above) not wanting to back a losing horse, also voting no); the best option offered the South was the Republican-backed idea of a national convention.[39]

Before the Peace Conference concluded its work, the president-elect held several meetings with various members, reaching out in particular to the Southern delegates. Of special significance to this story are Lincoln's interactions with Virginia Unionist William Rives, a former senator and U.S. Minister to France. Their interactions were cordial and Rives thought the president-elect was "good natured and well-intended." But when the subject turned to Fort Sumter, Rives told Lincoln that the fort "could not be relieved without the loss of thousands of lives, and to hold it was but a barren honor."

Lincoln first replied that if Virginia would pass a resolution barring secession, "I may then agree with you ... [that] a State any day is worth more than a fort."

When Rives responded that secession would result from coercive measures being taken by the federal government, Lincoln stood up and cried: "Mr. Rives! Mr. Rives! If Virginia will stay in, I will withdraw the troops from Fort Sumter."[40] [As we will see in Chapter IX, Lincoln (against Seward's advice) later (apparently) changed his mind about such a trade.][41]

Notes

1. Lincoln February 1, 1861, Letter to Seward (Roy Basler (ed.), *The Collected Works of Abraham Lincoln,* Volume 4, p. 183 (Rutgers University Press 1953-55)); see also Frederick W. Seward, *Seward at Washington: 1846-61,* p. 504 (Derby and Miller 1891).

2. Charles Francis Adams Diary (February 5, 1861) (Massachusetts Historical Society) (Seward added that Lincoln "was so badgered at Springfield that he felt compelled to keep uncommitted on it at present."). Harold Holzer well depicts the badgering Lincoln received from people seeking jobs in the new administration. Harold Holzer, *Lincoln President-Elect: Abraham Lincoln and the Great Secession Winter 1860-1861,* pp. 232-38 (Simon & Schuster 2008).

3. Walter Stahr's *Seward: Lincoln's Indispensable Man,* pp. 231-33 (Simon & Schuster 2012). Michael Burlingame wrote that Lincoln's "rather casual statement" regarding New Mexico "represented a momentous policy shift" by the president-elect; Burlingame further noted that the *Illinois State Journal* (a Lincoln house-organ) also seemed to endorsed the admission of New Mexico as a slave state (January 24, 1861). Michael Burlingame, *Abraham Lincoln: A Life,*

Volume I, pp. 749-50 (Johns Hopkins University Press 2009). He then wrote: "Lincoln's change of heart could perhaps have averted bloodshed if Seward had exploited it and if Southern Unionists had accepted the New Mexico scheme.... But nothing came of it, for Seward failed to act on Lincoln's new position regarding New Mexico statehood." Burlingame then concluded: "Seward's behavior is one of the great mysteries of the secession crisis." Id. p. 751. (Harold Holzer's take on Lincoln's February 1 letter to Seward is decidedly different—see Holzer, supra note 2, pp. 252-53 (calling it a "half-hearted gesture")).

But, as explained above in the text, Seward (obviously closer on the ground to the dynamics of power politics in Washington at this point than Lincoln) did not think that *any* plan would actually garner enough support to pass muster and he could not be seen as an outspoken advocate for a "rejected" plan. Daniel Crofts, *Reluctant Confederates: Upper South Unionists in the Secession Crisis*, pp. 242-43 (University of North Carolina Press 1987). That should not have been such a "mystery" to Michael Burlingame since he cited Lord Lyons's report to the British Home Office in that section of his book in which he is critical of Seward for his "dictator" comment to Mrs. Seward—see Burlingame, supra note 3, Volume I, p. 746) (see supra Chapter VI, note 1 (and text)). Burlingame omitted from his citation Lyons's statement that "[Seward] is sure that at this moment no plan would be accepted by both parties—and he does not choose to weaken his position by making himself responsible for a rejected plan." See supra Chapter VI note 5 (and accompanying text); see also Stahr, supra note 3, pp. 231-33.

4. A number of Northern Republicans were not enthused about the Peace Conference; "but Seward persuaded them to support the project as a gesture of good will." James McPherson, *Battle*

Cry of Freedom: The Civil War Era, p. 201 (Oxford University Press 1988).

5. Crofts, supra note 3, pp. 207-13; F. Seward, supra note 1, p. 503; Lawrence Denton, *William Henry Seward and the Secession Crisis*, p. 88 (McFarland & Company 2009).

6. Crofts, supra note 3, pp. 140-43 (Crofts provides a very helpful county-by-county analysis of the vote, which underscores the pro-Union bias of much of the state). Id. pp. 164-94, 361-81.

7. *New York Evening Post* (February 5 & 11, 1861); see Stahr, supra note 3, p. 234; Denton, supra note 5, p. 89; F. Seward, supra note 1, p. 502 ("At least the danger of conflict ... before the 4th of March has been averted. Time has been gained.").

8. Crofts, supra note 3, p. 142. For more analysis on Seward's thought process regarding a political party of moderates from the North and the Border States, see id. pp. 267-72; Denton, supra note 5, pp. 94-95, 106-07. See also Chapter VI supra note 5 (and accompanying text).

9. Crofts, supra note 3, pp. 144-52; Tennessee also voted for Unionist candidates to any convention vs. secession candidates by almost a 70,000 margin (approximately 100,000 to approximately 30,000). See id. p. 151 for a county-by-county breakdown of the Tennessee vote. Seward's reaction to Tennessee's vote was: "I think now that we shall go quietly into power on the 4th of March." F. Seward, supra note 1, p. 502. Maryland Congressman Henry Winter Davis believed that the two states' votes broke "the back of the revolution." Burlingame, supra note 3, Volume I, p. 751.

10. Adams February 8, 1861, letter to C.F. Adams Jr., *Letters of Henry Adams*, Volume I, p. 230 (J.C. Levenson ed.) (Harvard University Press 1982-1988); Stahr, supra note 3, pp. 234-35; Denton, supra note 5, p. 92. Seward was also said to have boasted:

> I have built up the Republican Party; I have brought it to triumph; but its advent to power is accomplished by great difficulties and perils. I must save the party and save the Government in its hands. To do this, war must be averted; the negro question dropped; the "irrepressible conflict" ignored; and a Union party to embrace the border slave states inaugurated. I have already whipped Mason and Hunter [Virginia's U.S. Senators] in their own state. I must crush out Davis and Toombs [Mississippi's just resigned U.S. Senators] and their colleagues in sedition in their respective states. Saving the border states to the Union by moderation and justice, the people of the cotton states, unwillingly led into secession, will rebel against their leaders, and reconstruction will follow.

Daniel Crofts, "Secession Winter: William Henry Seward and the Decision for War," *New York History* 245 (July 1984); Burlingame, supra note 3, Volume II, p. 99. Whether Seward ever said this (or anything like it) is *very* unclear. The source(s) of this quote are two of the three commissioners appointed by the Confederate government to get official recognition as a nation from the Federal government (see infra Chapter VIII). John Forsyth and Martin Crawford Dispatch No. 3 (dated March 8, 1861) to Robert Toombs (Confederate States of America Papers) (Library of Congress); see also Stahr, supra note 3, p. 260.

At the same time as Seward was in "high spirits" Lincoln was "exasperated" and downcast. While the Senate on January 21 had passed Seward's bill admitting Kansas as a free state (F. Seward, supra note 1, p. 498), on February 4, the Senate passed another bill organizing the Colorado Territory with no provision excluding slavery; similar legislation was subsequently enacted organizing Nevada and Dakota. Lincoln lamented to a close friend that Stephen Douglas had really won the 1860 election: "[M]y own party endorsed his popular sovereignty idea and applies it in legislation." Burlingame, supra note 3, Volume I, p. 758.

11. Lincoln January 3, 1861, letter to Seward (F. Seward, supra note 1, pp. 492-93).

12. Lincoln's circuitous trip is well documented in Ted Widmer's *Lincoln on the Verge: Thirteen Days to Washington* (Simon & Schuster 2020); see also Burlingame, supra note 3, Volume II, pp. 1-39; Holzer, supra note 2, pp. 295-396.

13. Widmer, supra note12, pp. 134-35. Burlingame terms this the "Hard-Line Speech in Indianapolis" (supra note 3, Volume II, pp. 4-7). Lincoln also segued into a risque exposition on "free love" versus traditional marriage (in the context of secession vs. union)—this was (to put it mildly) unprecedented public discourse for that time. Burlingame sets forth a representative sampling of the Southern press's critical reporting on Lincoln's "retaking" comment. Id. For understanding Lincoln's anger regarding Buchanan's allowing the seceding states to seize federal property ("they ought to hang him!"), see Burlingame, supra note 3, Volume I, pp. 754-55.

14. Widmer, supra note 12, pp. 184-86. Burlingame terms this the "Unfortunate Speech in Columbus" (supra note 3, Volume II, pp. 10-12). Critics, both North and South, attacked the president-elect's cluelessness that "nothing" had gone "wrong." Id.

15. Widmer, supra note 12, pp. 227-29. Burlingame terms this the "embarrassing speech in Pittsburgh" (supra note 3, Volume II, pp. 11-15). The Northern press particularly took issue with Lincoln's remarks. Id. pp. 19-23. See also Widmer, supra note 12, pp. 275-76.

16. His receptions by the snooty and politically heterogeneous crowds in New York City, however, were far from smooth. Not for the first (or last) time, Lincoln's physicality shocked many people. Widmer, supra note 12, pp. 321-49; Burlingame, supra note 3, Volume II, pp. 26-30. (He "is making an ass of himself.... [It is] disquieting, and exceedingly humiliating ... that we have become so degenerate, as to forward an obscure *ignoramus* like the President-Elect—to the highest position in the known world.")

17. Widmer, supra note 12, pp. 364-72. When he was finally able to continue, Lincoln asked: "And if I do my duty, and do right, you will sustain me, will you not?" That brought further cheers and cries of "Yes," "Yes," "We will." James McPherson, *Tried by War: Abraham Lincoln as Commander in Chief*, p. 12 (Penguin Press 2008). Burlingame terms this the "Resuming the Hard-Line Stance" (supra note 3, Volume II, pp. 30-32).

18. David Potter, *Lincoln and His Party in the Secession Crisis*, pp. 242-47, 317-18 (Louisiana State University Press 1995 (originally Yale University Press 1942)); Patrick Sowle, "The Conciliatory Republicans During the Winter of Secession," pp. 401-05 (Ph.D. Dissertation) (Duke University 1963); Crofts, "Secession Winter," supra note 10, p. 247 and *Reluctant Confederates*, supra note 3, pp. 243-44.

19. One of Seward's Virginia Unionists bemoaned: "We are struggling here against every obstacle, and Mr. Lincoln, by his speech in the North, has done vast harm. If he will not be guided by Mr. Seward but puts himself in the hands of Mr. Chase and the ultra Republicans, nothing can save the cause of the Union in the South." Frederick Bancroft, *The Life of William H. Seward*, Volume 2, p. 536 (Harper & Row 1900).

20. Charles Francis Adams February 18, 1861, letter to Richard Henry Dana (Dana Family Papers, Massachusetts Historical

Society); Charles Francis Adams February 21, 1861, Diary entry (Adams Family Papers, Massachusetts Historical Society); Charles Francis Adams Jr., *Charles Francis Adams, 1935-1915: An Autobiography*, p. 22 (Houghton Mifflin 1916); Charles Francis Adams Jr. February 22, 1861, letter to John Andrew (Andrew Papers, Massachusetts Historical Society); Charles Francis Adams Jr. February 21, 1861, letter to Richard Dana Jr. (Dana Papers, Massachusetts Historical Society). See also Burlingame, supra note 3, Volume II, pp. 19-20; Crofts, supra note 3, pp. 243-44; Stahr, supra note 3, pp. 236-37; Denton, supra note 5, p. 93.

21. See Widmer, supra note 12, pp. 249-50, Denton, supra note 5, p. 98, and Burlingame, supra note 3, Volume II, pp. 19-22 for a sampling of the widespread negative reaction(s) to Lincoln's railroad speeches.

22. A prior possible crisis (about which both Lincoln and Seward had expressed concern)—whether the Electoral College vote on February 13 would take place without incident—had been averted, with a significant assist by Seward (and General Winfield Scott). F. Seward, supra note 1, pp. 504-05; Widmer, supra note 12, pp. 190-94; Stahr, supra note 3, pp. 235-36; Denton, supra note 5, p. 94. Seward wrote to his wife on February 15: "We have passed the 13th safely.... I am, at last, out, of direct responsibility. I have brought the ship off the sands, and am ready to resign the helm into the hands of the Captain whom the people have chosen." (F. Seward, p. 505); Stahr, p. 236. Citing this letter, Burlingame grudgingly gives "credit" to Seward's efforts to this point for "manag[ing] to keep the Upper South in the Union, at least temporarily" (supra note 3, Volume I, p. 752).

23. Frederick Seward's accounts of the assassination episode are in Frederick Seward, *Reminiscence of a War-Time Statesman and*

Diplomat, 1830-1915, pp. 134-35 (G.P. Putnam's Sons 1916) and F. Seward, supra note 1, pp. 508-11. For other accounts, see Stahr, supra note 3, pp. 237-38; Widmer, supra note 12, pp. 379-81, 415-30; Burlingame, supra note 3, Volume II, pp. 32-37; Denton, supra note 5, pp. 98-99.

24. On that same day, Texas voters ratified the decision to secede 46,129 to 14,697. Five days earlier, Jefferson Davis had been sworn in as Provisional President of the Confederate States of America in Montgomery, Alabama.

25. In a February 23 letter to his wife, Seward wrote that he met Lincoln at the train station (F. Seward, supra note 1, p. 511); but by most accounts Seward met the group shortly after they arrived at the hotel. Stahr, supra note 3, p. 238; Burlingame, supra note 3, Volume II, p. 37. What is not in doubt is that Lincoln caught a lot of criticism for "sneaking" into Washington. Burlingame, supra note 3, Volume II, pp. 38-39; Widmer, supra note 12, p. 431.

26. David Donald, *Lincoln*, p. 281 (Simon & Schuster 1996); Stahr, supra note 3, pp. 238-39; Denton, supra note 5, pp. 100-03; Burlingame, supra note 3, Volume II, p. 45. On the evening of February 23, Lincoln said to Seward: "One part of the business, Governor Seward, I think I shall leave entirely in your hands; that is the dealing with those foreign nations and their governments." In his memoir, Frederick Seward remembered Lincoln's comment differently: "There is one part of my work that I shall have to leave largely to you. I shall have to depend upon you for taking care of these matters of foreign affairs, of which I know so little and which I reckon you are familiar." Frederick Seward, supra note 23, p. 147. See also Stahr, supra note 3, pp. 252-53.

It also appears that, at some point that same day, Lincoln gave Seward a draft of his Inaugural Address and asked for comments.

27. Crofts, supra note 3, pp. 245-47 (Gilmer was also upset after reading the hard-line text of the Inaugural Address Lincoln had written in Springfield and carried to Washington). Gilmer's decision came at the same time (February 28) that North Carolina was rejecting secession by a vote of 47,323 to 46,672 (and of the 120 delegates chosen for the state convention only 39 were secessionists). Id. pp. 144-52 (see also pp. 166, 169, 173, 180-82, 190 for analysis of North Carolina's 1861 voting). For Seward and Weed's unhappiness regarding the ultimate composition of the Cabinet, see Denton, supra note 5, pp. 102-04; Stahr, supra note 3, pp. 243-44.

28. Henry Adams, "The Great Secession Winter of 1860-61," p. 683, *Proceedings of the Massachusetts Historical Society* (1910). For the Southern Unionists' despondency regarding Chase's appointment, see Crofts, supra note 3, pp. 252-23.

29. See supra note 26; see also Stahr, supra note 3, p. 239. For Lincoln's work on the draft in Springfield, see Burlingame, supra note 3, Volume I, pp. 756-59.

30. There is, in fact, scholarly debate over the exact number of Seward's proposed changes. See Stahr, supra note 3, p. 239 ("more than fifty") versus Ronald White Jr., *The Eloquent President: A Portrait of Lincoln Through His Words*, p. 69 (Random House 2005) (forty-nine).

31. See supra Chapter IV, note 8. And, to a lesser extent, his February 29, 1860, Senate speech. See supra Chapter VI, notes 9-11 (and accompanying text).

32. F. Seward, supra note 1, pp. 512-13.

Many (pro-Lincoln) historians have been bemused by the purported self-important claims put forward by Seward in his February 24 letter to Lincoln (e.g., Potter, supra note 18, pp. 310-14). But given the significance of the Inaugural Address to the issue of a civil war (where over 700,000 people would ultimately die), this was hardly a time for false modesty. As even Potter acknowledges, Seward's vanity was "not without cause" (Id.; see also Bancroft, supra note 19, Volume 2, pp. 37-38; Crofts, supra note 10, p. 239); indeed, Seward's statement regarding his knowledge of events and key players was, in fact, true. As Dizzy Dean once said: "It ain't bragging if you can do it" (Quora) [See also Babe Ruth: "It's not Bragging if You can Really do it." Id.; Yogi Berra: "It Ain't Bragging If It's True." Id.]

The prior day Seward had written a letter to the editor of the *New York Independent*, revealing his motivation: "Twelve years ago freedom was in danger and the Union was not.... Today, ... freedom is not in danger, and Union is.... Now, therefore, I speak singly for the Union.... For this singleness of speech I am now suspected of infidelity to freedom.... I refer myself not to the men of my time, but to the judgment of history." John M. Taylor, *William Henry Seward: Lincoln's Right Hand*, p. 158 (HarperCollins 1991).

33. Lincoln's original sentence on this critical point was: "All the power at my disposal will be used to reclaim the public property and places which have fallen, to hold, occupy and possess these, and all other property and places belonging to the government, and to collect the duties on imports, but beyond what may be necessary for these objects, there will be no invasion of any State." In the address delivered on March 4 that sentence became: "The power confided in me, will be used to hold, occupy and possess the property, and places belonging to the government, and to collect the duties and imposts; but beyond what may be necessary for these objects, there will be no invasion—no using of force against or among the people anywhere." It is easy to see how the first version dissuaded Gilmer from joining the Cabinet (and how, if it had been delivered on March 4, Seward's

prediction of losing the Border States within weeks or months would have come to pass).

34. "In your hands, my dissatisfied fellow countrymen, and not in mine, is the momentous issue of civil war. The government will not assail you, unless first you assail it. You can have no conflict, without being yourselves the aggressors. You have no oath registered in Heaven to destroy the government, while I shall have the most solemn one to 'preserve, protect and defend' it. With you, and not with me, is the solemn question of 'shall it be peace, or a sword?'"

35. Stahr, supra note 3, pp. 240-41; Holzer, supra note 2, pp. 440-44; Burlingame, supra note 3, Volume II, pp. 45-51. See also Russell McClintock, *Lincoln and the Decision for War,* pp. 190-98 (University of North Carolina Press 2008); Douglas Wilson, *Lincoln's Sword: The Presidency and the Power of Words,* pp. 42-70 (Alfred Knopf 2006).

36. Crofts, supra note 3, p. 247 ("Lincoln ... gave no indication that he intended to modify the Inaugural Address. The original hard-lined text remained the official statement of Lincoln's views as Inauguration Day approached."); see also Stahr, supra note 3, p. 241.

37. Burlingame, supra note 3, Volume II, pp. 52-58; Stahr, supra note 3, pp. 241-42; Holzer, supra note 2, pp. 430-34; Glyndon Van Deusen, *William Henry Seward* , p. 251 (Oxford University Press 1967).

38. Crofts, "Reluctant Confederates," pp. 208-14, 248-51; Burlingame, supra note 3, Volume II, pp. 40-45.

39. Crofts, supra note 3, pp. 251-52; Denton, supra note 5, pp. 104-05; McPherson, supra note 4, pp. 200-01. Also endorsed was a call for stricter enforcement of the Fugitive Slave Law and repeal of the Northern personal liberty laws. James Barbour, one of the Virginia Unionists with whom Seward had worked closely over

the past several months, concluded that he had been stabbed in the back by Seward and warned his Virginia colleagues not to be further deceived by "one of the shrewdest and smartest men in this Union." (quoted in Crofts's *Reluctant Confederates*, supra note 3, p. 251).

Nonetheless, on February 28, a very fragile coalition of Southerners, Northern Democrats, and just enough conciliatory Republicans did get the House of Representatives to pass by a bare two-thirds majority (132 to 65) the Thirteenth Amendment proposed by Charles Francis Adams; it guaranteed perpetual protection of slavery in the states. Crofts, supra note 3, pp. 249-50.

40. Mark Tooley, *The Peace That Almost Was: The Forgotten Story of the 1861 Peace Conference and the Final Attempt to Avert the Civil War*, pp. 235-38 (Nelson Books 2015); Burlingame, supra note 3, Volume II, pp. 41-44; see also David Barbee & Milledge Bonham Jr. (eds.), "Fort Sumter Again," *Mississippi Valley Historical Review* 28 (1941); Potter, supra note 18, pp. 353-54; McPherson, supra note 17, p. 14.

41. Henry Adams would later make this observation about Seward's efforts to save the Union up to this point:

> Those who saw and followed Mr. Seward during all the anxieties and cares of this long struggle ... would not likely forget his cheerfulness, his steadfastness, his clear perception, his inexhaustible resourcefulness, his unfading tact, his influence in guiding the actions of others, his power of bringing diverse connections into a vast combination, his promptness in abandoning unattainable objectives, and his pertinacity in seeing as much as practicable. With all this "armory of weapons," he fought, during these three months of chaos, a fight

> which might go down in history as one of the wonders of statesmanship.

Adams, supra note 28, p. 679; Potter, supra note 18, pp. 278-79, 310-14; Bancroft, supra note 19, Volume 2, pp. 37-38 (Seward's efforts pre-March 4, 1861, were the supreme achievement of his public life and his principal claim to historical greatness).

Chapter VIII

March 1861—A New Administration

For Seward, March started off in a way that historians are still debating. Having heard nothing from Lincoln about whether the Inaugural Address would shift from confrontation to conciliation (and still upset about the no-compromise additions to the Cabinet, as well as John Gilmer's refusal to serve), Seward sent Lincoln a brief note on March 2: "Circumstances which have occurred since I expressed to you in December last my willingness to accept the office of Secretary of State seem to me to render it my duty to ask you to withdraw that consent."[1] With the Peace Convention having come up with nothing more than a slightly revised version of the Crittenden Compromise (which had failed) and an inaugural address (in his view) sure to cause the Upper

South to leave the Union, Seward was telling Lincoln he could not be part of a hard-line, aggressive administration, especially in light of everything Lincoln had been doing since the election.[2]

When Seward heard Lincoln's address on March 4, however, it was obvious that many of his changes had been adopted and the speech was much more conciliatory in substance and tone. Gone were the hard-line threats to re-take federal property.[3] Instead, Lincoln endorsed the just passed Thirteenth Amendment (by the Senate at 5 a.m. on March 4); he also promised to vigorously enforce the Fugitive Slave Law (citing to its constitutional antecedent). And, of course, Lincoln's famous closing lifted heavily from the Seward draft:

> I am loth [sic] to close—we are not enemies, but friends. We must not be enemies.
>
> Though passion may have strained, it must not break our bonds of affection. The mythic chords of memory, stretching from every battlefield and patriot grave, to every living heart and hearthstone, all over this broad land, will yet swell the chorus of the Union, when again touched, as surely this will be, by the better angels of our nature.[4]

Before giving his Inaugural Address, Lincoln had written to Seward asking him to reconsider his withdrawal. Meeting with Lincoln at the White House that afternoon, Seward agreed to Lincoln's request; and the next morning he confirmed in writing that he had yielded to the "opinion and wishes" expressed by the president.[5]

With the administration now in place, Seward began to take charge of the State Department, which was located in a not very elegant building near the White House (at Fifteenth Street and Pennsylvania Avenue). And although Lincoln had assured Seward almost unilateral authority in the conduct of foreign affairs (his first order of business was to install his son, Frederick, as assistant secretary of state—the number two job in the department),[6] the new Secretary of State had to dicker with the president on the selection of American ministers to major foreign capitals.[7] On some of these Seward had to yield to political debts Lincoln had to pay (for example, Norman Judd—who had first ensured that Chicago would be the site of the Republican Committee, and then later helped to pack the Wigwam with Lincoln supporters holding fake tickets—was given the post to Germany)[8]; most important to Seward (and later to the critical issue of preventing England from recognizing the Confederacy as an independent

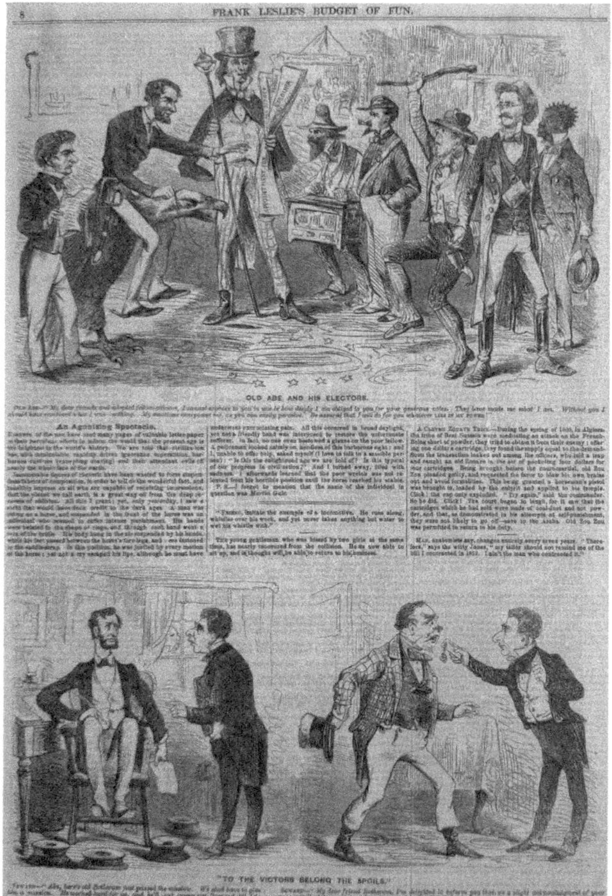

Frank Leslie's Budget of Fun
(Old Abe and His Electors; "To the Victors Belong the Spoils")
(published March 1861) (author's collection)

nation-state) was that the president yielded to Charles Francis Adams becoming the Ambassador to the Court of St. James.[9]

Seward's patronage issues were nothing compared to Lincoln's. The president, who felt besieged by office seekers while he was in Springfield, was completely underwater on that front in Washington—for example, on just one day alone (March 6) 1,000 job hunters descended upon the White House.[10] With one Lincoln biographer terming this "the engulfing tide of office seekers,"[11] Lincoln told Henry Raymond (the editor of the *New York Times*) in late March 1861 that "he wished he could get time to attend to the Southern question.... I am like a man so busy in letting rooms in one end of his house, that he can't stop to put out the fire that is burning the other."[12]

Fort Sumter (Part I)

Lincoln had deleted "reclaim" from his inaugural address, but he had publicly vowed to "hold, occupy and possess the property, and places belonging to the government" on March 4.[13] Upon becoming President, however, Lincoln learned from General Winfield Scott that Fort Sumter would be running out of supplies shortly, that resupply would be difficult or impossible, that any defense against attack would require 25,000 troops and a naval fleet, and that Scott saw "no alternative" except to surrender the fort. On December 7, the president shared this report with his Secretary of State.[14] At the second Cabinet meeting on March 9, the rest of the Cabinet was informed of the grim news about Sumter.[15]

Immediately, leaks abounded in the press that Sumter would be evacuated, and Scott drew up evacuation orders for Major Robert Anderson.[16] The leaks led to a prompt and fevered backlash among no-compromise Republicans, for whom Fort Sumter (especially since it had been fired upon in January) had taken on a tremendous symbolic value in the North (it had taken on an equal, but different symbolic value in the South—especially for the fire-eaters in South Carolina).[17]

On March 15, the President assembled his Cabinet again to hear and discuss what options were available to deal with the Sumter crisis. Gustavus Fox, a former naval officer (whose main qualification for attending the meeting was that he was Montgomery Blair's brother-in-law), told the Cabinet that a night-time re-supply mission might be possible. General Scott reiterated his (and the U.S. Army's) prior views about the practicalities and wisdom of any such course of action. At the conclusion of those presentations Lincoln asked all of his Cabinet officers to reply, in writing, to this question: "Assuming it to be possible to now provision Fort Sumpter [sic], under all the circumstances, is it wise to attempt it?"[18]

Seward immediately provided a detailed response to the President.[19] While the Border States "at the present moment, indicate a disposition to adhere to the Union, … they do so uneasily." Any attempt to resupply Fort Sumter would be viewed by those states as "coercion" of the seceded states, and that would push the Border States out of the Union (and lead to a civil war). Why risk a civil war over a fort that was indefensible and militarily (and strategically) unimportant? Non-action and delay were the best options, allowing for the "blinding unreasoning popular excitement" to abate, and for "devotion to the Union" to rise again in the South. Finally, Seward argued that any force used by the federal government should be defensive in nature. The first blows (if any) should come from "those who seek to dismember and subvert this Union"; by that policy "we should have the spirit of the country and the approval of mankind on our side."

Virtually all of the other Cabinet officers agreed with Seward's opposition to resupplying/reinforcing Fort Sumter, with only Montgomery Blair (strongly) disagreeing.[20]

After the Cabinet had weighed in, Lincoln urged his principal advisors to do nothing to foment further problems with the Border States, while he sought more information on whether anything could in fact be done for Major Anderson and his beleaguered men.[21]

Seward's Focus on Virginia

Seward, apparently believing the resupply issue was now resolved by the Cabinet vote (and also believing Lincoln's representations to him about conciliating the Border States), took the president at his word. In actuality, since the inauguration and the onset of his new duties as Secretary of State, Seward had not ceased in his efforts to (1) give support and encouragement to key Southern Union leaders (e.g., John Gilmer (of North Carolina) and George Summers (of Virginia)), and (2) underwrite in every way possible a political realignment in the Border States based on one issue: Union versus dis-Union.[22] Seward was strategically focused on the upcoming Virginia elections in May, where Union-loyal men hoped for a clean sweep; that, in Seward's view, would be "the decisive point," ensuring the basis for an (ultimate) peaceful resolution of the crisis.[23] He had bought time from November to March; could his luck hold out for two more months?

Between March 7 and 12, Gilmer sent Seward *four* letters, giving him a steady flow of intel on the nature of

Union versus dis-Union sentiment in the South. Gilmer warned Seward that the Fire-Eaters wanted "some collision of arms"; Gilmer also told him that if Sumter were not abandoned "as quickly as possible," and instead the fort triggered armed conflict, "the Conservative Union men in the border slave states ... will be swept away in a torrent of madness."[24]

At the same time that Seward was receiving this intel from Gilmer (and many others), he was also having to deal with three commissioners sent to Washington by Jefferson Davis. Their task was to have the federal government recognize the Confederacy as an independent nation.[25] Seeking an audience with Seward, the commissioners put the federal government in a tricky position—just having such a meeting would be the start of a slippery slope to recognition. Seward (and Lincoln) recognized this danger and decided to delay a "formal" rebuff as long as possible: the commissioners (although they had threatened to have Fort Sumter attacked if their audience was not granted) actually favored delay as well—every extra day allowed the Confederate government to get more established (both in Montgomery, Alabama, *and* in the eyes of European governments).[26]

Supreme Court Justice John Campbell became the three commissioners' back-channel to Seward; on the same day as the March 15 Cabinet meeting, he visited Seward at the State Department.[27] In response to a renewed request for at least a meeting (if not recognition itself), Seward is said to have replied: "There is not a member of the cabinet who would consent to it. If Jefferson Davis had known the state of things here, he would not have sent those commissioners. The evacuation of Sumter is as much as the administration can bear."[28]

That last comment immediately caught Campbell's ear. Could he report that to Jefferson Davis? ("And what should I say to him?") Seward's purportedly replied: "You may say to him that before that letter reaches him—how far is it to Montgomery? ["Three days," answered Campbell.] You may say to him that before the letter reaches him, the telegraph will have informed him that Sumter will have been evacuated."[29]

Seward went beyond Justice Campbell with this evacuation news. He used at least two men as conduits to inform George Summers that the federal government would soon abandon Fort Sumter. Summers reported back that the news had worked "like a charm," and had given Union men in Virginia (whose convention was still in session) "great strength": "We are masters of our position here, and can maintain it if left alone."[30] Seward also leaked to his friends in the New York press that the fort—indefensible and of no strategic or military value—would soon be evacuated.[31]

One important question unresolved by historians is whether Seward was acting on his own, or with the president's explicit (or implicit) approval. Frederick Seward left no record on this score. Lincoln's aides, John Nicolay and John Hay, years later wrote that Seward thought he was speaking for the administration and "undoubtedly believed every word of this at the moment."[32]

What we *do know* is that one of the individuals Seward used as a conduit to George Summers was New York Congressman John Cochrane. On March 19, Seward arranged for Cochrane to meet with the president to report on his missions. In his letter of introduction (telling Lincoln that Cochrane was someone with whom he could "converse freely"), Seward told Lincoln that the congressman had just received "a noble letter from Summers, which was written upon explanations made to him by Mr. Cochrane from me."[33] The "noble letter" has (apparently) not survived, but a copy of another letter written by Summers that same day has survived; it expressly references the fact that Seward's assurances of Sumter's evacuation had strengthened the hand of Virginia Union leaders.[34] As such, by March 19 (if not before), Lincoln was fully aware of what Seward had "pledged" regarding the fate of Fort Sumter.[35]

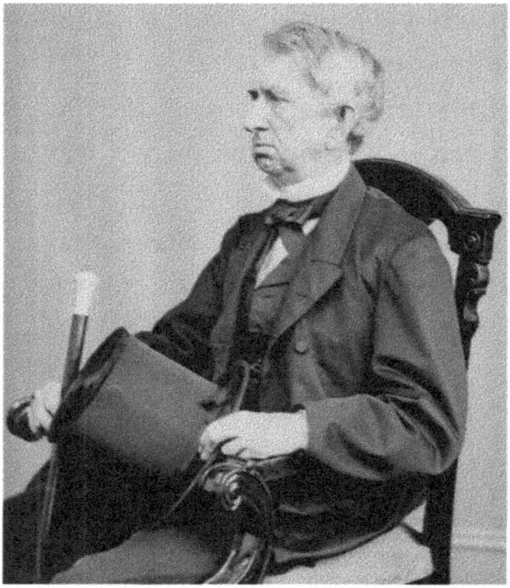

William Henry Seward
(Lincoln's Secretary of State)
(author's collection)

Lincoln's Fact-Finding

Nonetheless, still beleaguered by patronage seekers, and under attack for seeming "to be playing 'shilly shally,' one day one way the next other way …, permit[ing] the Courageous & Chivaric South to spit on you, & walk over you, & kick you, and do just as they d[am]n please with you,"[36] Lincoln—to buy more time—took what historians have called (with a fair amount of understatement) an "unconventional" step[37]: he sent three men to Charleston, South Carolina, to assess the state of play in the belly of the fire-eating beast.

The three men selected did not bode well for the mission. Gustavus Fox (the advocate of resupplying Fort Sumter) was sent to assess the military situation. Stephen Hurlbut (an Illinois lawyer who Lincoln knew; he had been born in Charleston), and Ward Hill Lamon (Lincoln's bodyguard) were sent to "sample public opinion."[38]

Hurlbut reported back that (no surprise) Union sentiment was nonexistent in Charleston. He also reported that the South Carolina militia had a vast supply of batteries, and it was the militia's "intention to reduce the fort at all hazards."

Lamon's work in Charleston was of a different character. He told both Anderson *and* South Carolina Governor Francis Pickens that Sumter would be evacuated in short order (and that his mission was "to facilitate" the evacuation).[39]

Fox, who was a true believer as to his ability to lead a naval force into Charleston Harbor to resupply the beleaguered fort, did not come away from his visit dissuaded. Rather, he continued to hold on to that view even *after* Anderson told him (1) such an effort could never evade the harbor batteries, and (2) such an effort would trigger a civil war. Knowing that he had not convinced the gung ho Fox of the folly of his intentions, Anderson also sent a strongly worded report to the War Department about the absolute folly of any re-supply mission.[40]

As the "fact-finding" for the president played out, his Secretary of State was trying to juggle several balls at once. Justice Campbell (on behalf of the commissioners) impatiently asked why (after the "three days" had passed) there had been no news of evacuation; Seward advised patience, all would be well. At the same time, William Russell, a correspondent for *The Times* (of London), was told by Seward: "We will give up nothing that we have—abandon nothing that has been entrusted to us." And Russia minister Edouard de Stoeckl was being told that the seceding states "would be permitted to depart in peace," but the Secretary of State needed more time because of domestic political issues.[41]

On top of all of the foregoing, on March 25, at a dinner party hosted by British minister Lord Richard Lyons, the subject of the Federal Government interdicting ships leaving Southern ports without the necessary (U.S.) papers gave rise to a heated debate. Lyons stated that such action might well constitute a blockade [a violation of international law] and thus would place foreign governments "in the dilemma of recognizing the Southern Confederation or of submitting to the interruption of their commerce" [i.e., cotton]. The threat of European recognition of Jefferson Davis's government triggered an angry (for Seward) and lengthy response—the Secretary of State knew that, if there were such recognition, successful reunification of the country would be impossible.[42]

Fort Sumter (Part II)

Lincoln reconvened his cabinet officers at the White House on March 29. The prior night General Scott had given Lincoln a memorandum calling for the evacuation of Fort Sumter *and* (for the first time) Fort Pickens "to give confidence to the eight remaining slave-holding states now wavering between adherence to the Union and secession." Lincoln's leading biographer, David Donald, called this memorandum (with good reason) "shocking advice."[43] Lincoln was enraged by the General's new recommendation (as well as his seeming to step across the line into the realm of political advice).[44]

Why add Fort Pickens to the property to be evacuated by the federal government? The fort was a mile and a half off-shore Pensacola, Florida; it was militarily defensible and had strategic value for purposes of controlling coastal traffic; it was well-supplied and protected by a naval fleet; and it did not have the symbolic importance of Fort Sumter to the South (sitting smack dab in the middle of Charleston Harbor).

Before getting Scott's memorandum, the president had himself concluded that, if he evacuated Sumter, "he would justify it as a matter of practical necessity while simultaneously asserting federal authority by reinforcing Fort Pickens." And this was not just "what if" thinking—Lincoln had already told three Republican congressmen of his planned trade-off. But now Scott's ill-timed advice changed the decision-making dynamics.[45]

After hearing Fox's optimistic report on his "workable" plan (and seeing how angry Lincoln was at Scott's memorandum), the Cabinet secretaries began to change their minds on resupplying Sumter. Gideon Welles now joined Montgomery Blair, and Salmon Chase went from equivocal to non-equivocal (i.e., support). Edward Bates supported reinforcing Pickens, but equivocated on Sumter. Only Seward and Caleb Smith recommended evacuating Sumter, and reinforcing Pickens.[46] As to Sumter, Seward warned: "I do not think it wise to provoke a civil war beginning at Charleston and in rescue of an untenable position."[47] But trying to stay standing while the ground was shifting beneath his feet, Seward now advised Lincoln to "prepare for a war at Pensacola and Texas, to be taken however only as a consequence of maintaining the possessions and authority of the United States."[48] And while Seward turned his attention to a plan to resupply Fort Pickens, Lincoln sent Fox to New York, "with verbal directions to prepare for the voyage to Sumter."[49]

After the Cabinet meeting, Seward sought out Army Captain Montgomery Meigs, who was an engineer supervising work on the U.S. Capitol; more importantly, Meigs had just visited Fort Pickens. Seward brought the captain to meet with the president; at the meeting Meigs told Lincoln that Fort Pickens was eminently defensible. Between that meeting and Sunday afternoon (Easter Sunday, March 31), Seward, Meigs, and Erasmus Keyes (an aide to General Scott) worked up a Fort Pickens plan—under the State Department's authority; *not* the Navy Department's (because of concern that "some of the [Navy] clerks were known to be secessionists")—for the president's approval. Late that afternoon Lincoln approved the plan to resupply the fort: "I depend upon you gentlemen to push the thing through."[50]

Notes

1. Seward March 2, 1861, letter to Lincoln (Lincoln Papers, Library of Congress); see also Walter Stahr, *Seward: Lincoln's Indispensable Man*, pp. 243-44 (Simon & Schuster 2012).

2. There are two schools of thought about Seward's March 2 letter—both believe it was a "bluff." Starting with John Nicolay and John Hay's "Abraham Lincoln: A History: The Formation of the Cabinet," *Century Magazine* 35 (1988) (see also Michael Burlingame, *Abraham Lincoln: A Life*, Volume II, pp. 56-58 (Johns Hopkins University Press 2009); Glyndon Van Deusen, *William Henry Seward*, pp. 253-54 (Oxford University Press 1967)), the traditional view is that it was a "bluff" called triumphantly by Lincoln; his aides quoted their boss—who ultimately got Seward to change his mind—as saying "I can't afford to let Seward take the first trick." Other scholarship (more compelling in my view) believes it was a "bluff" successfully used by Seward to cause Lincoln to significantly soften the language of his inaugural address and have the president-elect take conciliatory steps vis-à-vis the Border States after being inaugurated. Daniel Crofts, *Reluctant Confederates: Upper South Unionists in the Secession Crisis*, p. 254 (University of North Carolina Press 1987), and "Secession Winter: William Henry Seward and the Decision for War," *New York History*, pp. 249-50 (1984); Russell McClintock, *Lincoln and the Decision for War*, pp. 190-99 (University of North Carolina Press 2008); Patrick Sowle, "The Conciliatory Republicans During the Winter of Secession," pp. 448-49(Ph.D. Dissertation) (Duke University 1963); Stahr, supra note 1, pp. 243-45; Lawrence Denton, *William Henry Seward and the Secession Crisis*, pp. 114-16 (McFarland & Company 2009).

3. See supra Chapter VII, note 33.

4. Roy Basler (ed.), *The Collected Works of Abraham Lincoln*, Volume 4, p. 271 (Rutgers University Press 1953-55); Don Fehrenbacher (ed.), *Abraham Lincoln, Speeches and Writing*, Volume 2, p. 224 (Library of America 1989). Garry Wills has provided a comparative analysis of Seward's ending and Lincoln's re-write thereof in *Lincoln at Gettysburg: The Words That Remade America*, pp. 158-59 (Simon & Schuster 1992); see also Waldo Braden, *Abraham Lincoln: Public Speaker*, pp. 56-61 (Louisiana State University Press 1998).

5. Lincoln March 4, 1861, letter to Seward (Basler, supra note 4, Volume 4, p. 273); Seward March 5, 1861, letter to Lincoln (Lincoln Papers, Library of Congress); see also Weed March 7, 1861, letter to Seward (Seward Papers, University of Rochester). Two other sources suggest that Lincoln went out of his way to provide "assurances" to Seward regarding a conciliatory policy vis-à-vis the Border States (see Crofts, *Reluctant Confederates*, supra note 2, pp. 254-55 and "Secession Winter," supra note 2, p. 250). The first comes from Seward's March 8, 1861, letter to his wife:

> The President is determined that he will have a compound Cabinet; and that it shall be peaceful, and even permanent. I was at one time on the point of refusing—nay, I did refuse, for a time to hazard myself in the experiment. But a distracted country appeared before me; and I withdrew from that position. I believe I can endure as much as any one; and may be that I can endure enough to make the experiment successful. At all events I did not dare to go home, or to England [as U.S. Ambassador] and leave the country to chance.

Frederick W. Seward, *Seward at Washington: 1846-61*, pp. 518-19 (Derby and Miller 1891).

The other source is Thurlow Weed's account to New York lawyer, John Bigelow, who recorded in his diary that Lincoln told Seward "he could not get on without his help and begged him to hold on." And after Seward rescinded his withdrawal, Lincoln "gave him to understand that whatever others might say or do, they two would not disagree but were friends." John Bigalow Diary, March 27, 1861 (New York Public Library); see also McClintock, supra note 2, p. 198; Stahr, supra note 1, p. 248; Denton, supra note 2, p. 116.

6. Frederick Seward, *Reminiscences of a War Time Statesman and Diplomat: 1830-1915*, pp. 139-43 (G.P. Putnam's Sons 1916). See supra Chapter VII, note 26; see also F. Seward, supra note 5, pp. 519-23; Van Deusen, supra note 2, pp. 269-74.

7. Stahr, supra note 1, pp. 253-56; F. Seward, supra note 5, pp. 524-25.

8. For Paris, Lincoln ultimately picked New Jersey Senator (and Fremont's 1856 running mate) William Dayton. Dayton, who was elderly and spoke no French, was not favored by Seward. However, Seward secured John Bigelow (a New York lawyer who was fluent in French, and a friend of his and Weed) to be appointed to the number-two post under Dayton. Stahr, supra note 1, pp. 254-55; John M. Taylor, *William Henry Seward: Lincoln's Right Hand*, p. 143 (HarperCollins 1991); Burlingame, supra note 2, Volume II, pp. 93-95.

9. Thanking Lincoln for his appointment, Adams was brusquely told by the president: "Very kind of you to say so, Mr. Adams, but you are not my choice. You are Seward's man." Taylor, supra note 8, p. 143; Denton, supra note 2, p. 129.

10. Burlingame, supra note 2, Volume II, p. 69; F. Seward, supra note 5, pp. 523-24.

11. Burlingame, supra note 2, Volume II, pp. 70-73, 75-93, 95-97.

12. Henry Raymond, *The Life and Public Services of Abraham Lincoln*, p. 720 (Derby and Miller 1865). On March 16, 1861, Seward wrote to his wife about Lincoln's preoccupation with just his patronage problems:

> This President proposes to do all his work. Of course he takes that business up, first, which is pressed upon him most. Solicitants for offices besiege him, and he, of course finds his hands full at present.

F. Seward, supra note 5, p. 530; see also Stahr, supra note 1, p. 258.

13. See supra Chapter VII, note 33 (and accompanying text).

14. F. Seward, supra note 5, p. 526; Crofts, *Reluctant Confederates*, supra note 2, pp. 274-75; Burlingame, Volume II, pp. 99-100. On March 3, Scott had sent Seward a letter containing similar information about Sumter; it rejected military means as a viable option to deal with secession, and urged a conciliatory policy to win back the wayward states. See *The Lincoln Papers*, Volume 2, pp. 456-57 (David Mearns ed.) (Doubleday 1948); Crofts terms this letter "an extraordinary document." *Reluctant Confederates*, supra note 2, p. 271; see also Burlingame, supra note 2, Volume II, p. 99. As he would later do that same month, Scott was mostly giving political advice; included was his suggestion that Lincoln's administration "assume a *new* designation—the Union Party" as the best way to peacefully (and successfully) deal with the secession crisis. Seward shared Scott's letter with Lincoln on March 4. Mearns (supra this note).

15. Most of the other Cabinet officers were shocked and disheartened by this report. Attorney General Bates, for example, wrote in his diary that he was "astounded" that the fort "must be

evacuated." *The Diary of Edward Bates, 1859-1866*, Volume 4, p. 177 (Howard Beale ed.) (U.S. Government Printing Office 1937); Stahr, supra note 1, p. 260; Burlingame, supra note 2, Volume II, p. 100.

16. Stahr, supra note 1, pp. 260-62; Burlingame, supra note 2, Volume II, pp. 100-01.

17. F. Seward, supra note 5, pp. 527-28; Burlingame, supra note 2, Volume II, pp. 100-04; Denton, supra note 2, pp. 122-26; Crofts, *Reluctant Confederates*, supra note 2, pp. 261-62 and "Secession Winter," supra note 2, p. 251. Weed promptly warned Seward that the "surrender of Fort Sumpter [sic] is to be [a] bitter thing for the [Northern] people." Weed March 12, 1861, letter to Seward (Seward Papers, University of Rochester).

18. Burlingame, supra note 2, Volume II, p. 102; Stahr, supra note 1, p. 261; see also Lincoln March 19, 1861, letter to Seward (Basler, supra note 4, Volume 4, p. 284). For some reason, Lincoln was never able to spell Sumter correctly. (Weed was similarly challenged.)

19. Seward March 15, 1861, Memorandum to Lincoln (Lincoln Papers, Library of Congress); F. Seward, supra note 5, pp. 528-29; Burlingame, supra note 2, Volume II, p. 101; Stahr, supra note 1, p. 261.

20. Burlingame, supra note 2, Volume II, pp. 102-03; Stahr, supra note 1, p. 261. Chase, it appears, offered Lincoln "yes" and "no" advice. Burlingame, supra note 2, Volume II, p. 102; James McPherson, *Trial by War: Abraham Lincoln as Commander in Chief*, p. 16 (Penguin Press 2008). Historians have tallied the Cabinet votes differently. Compare Van Deusen, supra note 2, p. 278 ("Blair and Chase said 'yes,' Smith wavered, but Seward and the rest said 'no.'") with Burlingame and McPherson (supra this note), Stahr, supra note 1, p. 261 ("only Blair disagreed"), and note 21 infra.

21. Burlingame, supra note 2, Volume II, p. 103. Years after the Civil War, Lincoln's aides John Nicolay and John Hay, wrote history (with the benefit of hindsight) this way:

> As requested, the members of the Cabinet returned somewhat elaborate replies, setting forth their reasons and conclusions. Two of the them, Chase and Blair, *agreeing with the President's own inclinations,* responded in the affirmative; the five others, Seward, Cameron, Welles, Smith[;] and Bates, advised against the measure. With his advisors divided, Lincoln was unable to reach a decision.

John Nicolay & John Hay, *Abraham Lincoln: A History,* Volume 3, p. 385 (emphasis added); see also Denton, supra note 2, p. 127. Weighing heavily on Lincoln was keeping the Republican Party unified and not conceding the legitimacy of the Confederacy. See Basler, supra note 4, Volume 4, pp. 288-90.

Contrary to Nicolay and Hay's decades-old memories, at the time Thurlow Weed insisted he had "conclusive evidence" that Lincoln had told three different men he would abandon Sumter if it meant keeping Virginia in the Union. Van Deusen, supra note 2, p. 278. See also supra Chapter VII, note 40 (and accompanying text).

22. Seward's pre-March efforts in these areas are set forth in Chapter VII, notes 5-10 (and accompanying text); his efforts in March 1861 are set forth above, but in even greater detail in Crofts, *Reluctant Confederates,* supra note 2, pp. 257-76.

23. Crofts, "Secession Winter," supra note 2, pp. 250-51; Denton, supra note 2, p. 125.

24. Gilmer's March 7, 8, and 12 letters to Seward are in the Seward Papers (University of Rochester); his letter of March 9 is

in the Lincoln Papers (Library of Congress). See also Crofts, *Reluctant Confederates*, supra note 2, pp. 257-59; F. Seward, supra note 5, pp. 527-28; Van Deusen, supra note 2, pp. 276-77. For other Southern feedback to Seward on this score, see North Carolinian, Frederick Robert's March 18, 1861, letter to Seward ("Once this unfortunate controversy produces a clash of arms, it will unite the whole South.") (Seward Papers, University of Rochester); see also Taylor, supra note 8, p. 154.

25. The three men were John Forsyth, Martin Crawford, and A.B. Roman. F. Seward, supra note 5, pp. 530-31; Van Deusen, supra note 2, pp. 278-79; Stahr, supra note 1, pp. 26-62; Denton, supra note 2, pp. 126-27. Jefferson Davis may have been emboldened to send these emissaries seeking such an extraordinary sanction because of back-channel messages he had received from his old friend, Seward, that the new administration "would be dependably conservative." William Baringer, *A House Dividing: Lincoln as President-Elect*, p. 322 (Abraham Lincoln Association 1945); David Potter, *Lincoln and His Party in the Secession Crisis*, pp. 343-44 (Louisiana State University Press 1995 (originally Yale University Press 1942)); Denton, supra note 2, p. 113; Burlingame, supra note 2, Volume II, p. 106.

26. Van Deusen, supra note 2, pp. 277-78; Denton, supra note 2, pp. 126-27; Burlingame, supra note 2, Volume II, p. 106; F. Seward, supra note 5, p. 531. At the same time, Seward (with Lincoln's approval) authored a confidential State Department "Memorandum" stating that secession was unconstitutional, the federal government would never recognize the seceded states as an independent nation, and the president would never meet with representatives of those states seeking recognition. The Memorandum is quoted at length in F. Seward, supra note 5, pp. 530-31.

27. Historians have differed as to whether Justice Campbell (from Alabama) acted alone as the intermediary or was joined by Justice Samuel Nelson (from New York). Compare Potter, supra note 25, pp. 345-47, with Burlingame, supra note 2, Volume II, pp. 106-07. Both Justices had concurred in Chief Justice Roger Taney's odious *Dred Scott* decision. See C. Evan Stewart, *The Worst Supreme Court Decisions, Ever! (And Related Tales)* (Chapter I) (Twelve Tables Press 2024). After the Civil War started, Campbell resigned from the Court (and later served the Confederacy as Assistant Secretary of War); Nelson served on the Court until 1872.

28. The quotations attributed to this meeting are from the commissioners' letters back to the Confederate Secretary of State (based on Campbell's de-briefings). Potter, supra note 25, pp. 345-46; Burlingame, supra note 2, Volume II, pp. 106-07.

29. Whether this was a "pledge" or "prediction" (see Burlingame, supra note 2, Volume II, pp. 106-07) is splitting hairs at an extremely high level. Clearly, Campbell, the commissioners, and the recipients of this message in Montgomery thought that the issue regarding Fort Sumter had been resolved.

30. Crofts, *Reluctant Confederates*, supra note 2, p. 275; Stahr, supra note 1, pp. 261-62; Denton, supra note 2, p. 130. Besides the good news from Virginia, Seward also heard that secession in Arkansas "was thus far, a failure"; and similar news had come in from Maryland, Kentucky, and Missouri. F. Seward, supra note 5, pp. 532-33.

31. Denton, supra note 2, p. 128; Burlingame, supra note 2, Volume II, pp. 107-08.

32. Nicolay & Hay, supra note 21, Volume 3, p. 408; see also Denton, supra note 2, p. 129.

33. Seward March 19, 1861, letter to Lincoln (Lincoln Papers, Library of Congress).

34. Summers March 19, 1861, letter to James Welling (Blair Family Papers, Library of Congress).

35. Crofts, *Reluctant Confederates*, supra note 2, p. 276; Denton, supra note 2, p. 130. At this same time Stephen Douglas was also in the picture helping Seward. On March 21, he introduced Seward to Virginia Unionist Alfred Barbour (of Harper's Ferry and a member of the convention at Richmond): "You can talk with him freely on the State of the Union and rely implicitly upon his discretion and honor." Douglas March 21, 1861, letter to Seward, *The Letters of Stephen A. Douglas*, p. 508 (Robert Johannsen ed.) (University of Illinois Press 1961).

36. Benjamin French April 5, 1861, letter to Frank French (French Family Papers, Library of Congress); see also Burlingame, supra note 2, Volume II, p. 104.

37. Burlingame, supra note 2, Volume II, p. 104.

38. Stahr, supra note 1, p. 262; Denton, supra note 2, p. 128; Burlingame, supra note 2, Volume II, pp. 104-06.

39. Rather than reporting to Lincoln, Lamon wrote to Seward that he was "satisfied of the policy and propriety of immediately evacuating Fort Sumpter [sic]." Lamon March 25, 1861, Letter to Seward (Seward Papers, University of Rochester). See also Burlingame, supra note 2, Volume II, p. 106.

40. Denton, supra note 2, pp. 132-35; Burlingame, supra note 2, Volume II, p. 105.

41. Stahr, supra note 1, pp. 265-66; Burlingame, supra note 2, Volume II, p. 107; Taylor, supra note 8, pp. 149-50.

42. Seward revisited the subject of European recognition with William Russell (*The Times* (of London) reporter) on March 27 at the State Department. Stahr, supra note 1, pp. 263-66; Van Deusen, supra note 2, pp. 288-89; Taylor, supra note 8, pp. 149-50. See also

Crofts, *Reluctant Confederates*, supra note 2, p. 285; Potter, supra note 25, p. 370; Burlingame, supra note 2, Volume II, p. 118.

43. David Donald, *Lincoln*, p. 288 (Simon & Schuster 1996).

44. Lincoln told Scott that following such recommendations would destroy his administration, and, if the General "could not carry out [Lincoln's orders], some other person might." McPherson, supra note 20, pp. 17-18; Crofts, *Reluctant Confederates*, supra note 2, pp. 296-97; Stahr, supra note 1, pp. 266-67; Burlingame, supra note 2, Volume II, p. 108; Denton, supra note 2, pp. 134-36. Some historians have speculated that Scott was "probably acting at the behest of Seward." Burlingame, supra note 2, Volume II, p. 308; Crofts, *Reluctant Confederates*, supra note 2, p. 293. While that might make sense given Scott and Seward's close relationship, there is no record evidence to support that speculation.

45. Potter, supra note 25, pp. 360-61; Burlingame, supra note 2, pp. 107-08; Crofts, *Reluctant Confederates*, supra note 2, pp. 296-97.

46. Simon Cameron was (inexplicably) absent for the March 29 meeting and did not weigh in on this matter.

47. Van Deusen, supra note 2, p. 279.

48. Seward March 29, 1861, Memorandum on Fort Sumter (Lincoln Papers, Library of Congress). In Texas, Governor Sam Houston was trying to hold off the forces of secession; ultimately, he declined Lincoln's offer to send federal troops. Burlingame, supra note 2, Volume II, p. 111; Stahr, supra note 1, p. 268; Crofts, *Reluctant Confederates*, supra note 2, p. 298.

49. F. Seward, supra note 5, p. 534; Stahr, supra note 1, p. 268; Crofts, *Reluctant Confederates*, supra note 2, p. 297. Lincoln's exact order was: "I desire that an expedition, to move by sea, be got ready to sail as early as the 6th of April next." Denton, supra note 2, p. 137.

50. Stahr, supra note1, pp. 268-69, 273-74; Burlingame, supra note 2, Volume II, pp. 112-13; F. Seward, supra note 5, p. 534. On April 1, Lincoln assured Seward and those assisting him that he would handle any "turf" issues that might arise with the Secretary of the Navy ("I think I can sooth the old fellow.").

Chapter IX

April 1861—And the War Came[1]

April Fool's Day 1861 was one of the busiest (and most consequential) days in the lead-up to the American Civil War. Knowing that the president had given Fox the order to resupply Fort Sumter (and thus likely to provoke the beginning of a war), Seward had another trick up his sleeve to stave off that war. After consulting with his friends and advisors, Thurlow Weed and Henry Raymond,[2] Seward wrote a document that has "puzzled and troubled [some] historians ever since it was first published in 1888 as part of the biography of Lincoln by his secretaries, John Nicolay and John Hay."[3] Because of this (purported) "puzzlement", and because of the document's importance, it is set forth in toto here:

Some Thoughts for the President's Consideration

April 1, 1861.

First. We are at the end of a month's administration and yet without a policy either domestic or foreign.

Second. This, however, is not culpable, and it has been unavoidable. The presence of the Senate, with the need to meet applications for patronage have prevented attention to other and more grave matters.

Third. But further delay to adopt and prosecute our policies for both domestic and foreign affairs would not only bring scandal on the administration, but danger upon the country.

Fourth. To do this we must dismiss the applicants for office. But how? I suggest that we make the local appointments forthwith, leaving foreign or general ones for ulterior and occasional action.

Fifth. The policy at home. I am aware that my views are singular, and perhaps not sufficiently explained. My system is built upon this idea as a ruling one, namely that we must

Change the question before the Public from one upon Slavery, or about Slavery for a question upon Union or Disunion.

In other words, from what would be regarded as a party question, to one of Patriotism or Union.

The occupation or evacuation of Fort Sumter, although not in fact a slavery or a party question, is so regarded. Witness the temper manifested by the Republicans in the free States, and even by the Union men in the South.

I would therefore terminate it as a safe means for changing the issue. I deem it fortunate that the last administration created the necessity.

For the rest, I would simultaneously defend and reinforce all the ports in the gulf, and have the navy recalled from foreign stations to be prepared for a blockade. Put the island of Key West under martial law.

This will raise distinctly the question of Union or Disunion. I would maintain every fort and possession in the South.

For Foreign Nations

I would demand explanations from Spain and France, categorically, at once.

I would seek explanations from Great Britain and Russia, and send agents into Canada, Mexico, and Central America to rouse a vigorous continental spirit of independence on this continent against European intervention.

And, if satisfactory explanations are not received from Spain and France,

Would convene Congress and declare war against them.

But whatever policy we adopt, there must be energetic prosecution of it.

For this purpose it must be somebody's business to pursue and direct it incessantly.

Either the President must do it himself, and be all the while active in it, or

Devolve it on some member of his cabinet. Once adopted, debates on it must end, and all agree and abide.

It is not in my especial province;

But I neither seek to evade nor assume responsibility.[4]

Notwithstanding the "puzzlement" of many historians regarding the Seward memorandum,[5] a small handful of historians—who tried to put themselves in Seward's shoes at the end of March 1861 (and thus not write history through the prism of 20-20 hindsight)—consider the document "readily comprehensible."[6] So, what actually was Seward trying to do, and why?? The best way to answer those questions is to break down the document into segments.

The first segment—which bluntly avers that the administration is "yet without a policy" (and thereafter explains why)—was perhaps unfortunate advocacy for purposes of persuading its audience of one; yet it was also true. The new and inexperienced president was totally consumed and overwhelmed by the patronage-hungry hordes descending upon him daily (and, as Lincoln himself explained to Henry Raymond, this had kept him from focusing on how to deal with the secession crisis). Moreover, beyond his total exhaustion from work and stress, the president was having trouble sleeping and at one point "keeled over" and suffered "one of his rare migraine headaches."[7]

The Northern press certainly agreed that the new administration did not seem to have an articulated policy for dealing with the crisis; some thought that was actually not a bad thing, while others (especially those representing the no-compromise wing of the Republican Party) expressed strong dissatisfaction that the federal government had not been more confrontational with the departed Southern states.[8] Furthermore, a wide spectrum of prominent politicos felt the same way about the new administration's non-policy as did Seward.[9]

With respect to the section of the document concerning "Change the question before the public from one upon Slavery, or about Slavery, for a question upon Union or Disunion," that could not possibly have been a surprise to the president. Seward had been publicly and privately urging this message repeatedly for months (including to the president-elect).[10] And that part of Seward's Southern Strategy had been demonstrably working. It had kept the Border States within the Union—to date; and it would continue to work (as will be seen on April 4), almost right up until the firing on Fort Sumter.

As for the de-linking of the need to resupply Fort Sumter *and* Fort Pickens, this is precisely what Lincoln had concluded was the best course of action—before General Scott's unfortunate recommendation of March 28.[11] Give up the indefensible fort (and the most important symbol to the South), while keeping the defensible fort (which was less of a symbolic stick in the

South's eye);[12] and taking the issue out of party politics, making it instead a question of "Patriotism or Union."[13]

The section captioned "For Foreign Nations" has drawn more attention (and criticism) from scholars. But this section was, in fact, written with important strategic goals in mind. Only days before there had been a revolution in the Caribbean on San Domingo (now the Dominican Republic); and the *New York Times* had just reported that Spain would be sending 5,000 troops to the island to reestablish it as a Spanish colony. There had also been reports that France was taking preliminary steps to exert influence (or something more) in Mexico.[14]

Of even greater concern was that some or all of the European governments might soon take steps to recognize the Confederacy.[15]

Since December of 1860, Seward had been publicly discussing using a foreign crisis to strengthen Union sentiment in both sections of the country,[16] so this idea was also not new. And besides reasserting the primacy of the Monroe Doctrine (authored by his hero, John Quincy Adams) to the European nations, holding onto Fort Pickens and demonstrating a strong naval presence in the Gulf of Mexico and the Caribbean (regardless of Sumter's fate) would make it clear to the Europeans that the federal government did not (and would not) agree or acquiesce to Southern secession and independence.[17]

As for some historians' belief that Seward was "in earnest" about wanting to fight a war against some/any European nation(s),[18] the best considered answer on that front is: "no". What Seward wanted was the "threat" of war to achieve a complex combination of domestic political goals *and* strategic geopolitical goals.[19] This was hardly "slap-dash improvisation."[20]

Lincoln composed an answer in writing the same day. His response is set forth below in toto.

Executive Mansion, April 1, 1861

Hon. W. H. Seward.

> My dear Sir: Since parting with you I have been considering your paper dated this day, and entitled "Some Thoughts for the President's Consideration." The first proposition in it, "*First,* We are at the end of a month's administration, and yet without a policy either domestic or foreign."
>
> At the beginning of that month, in the inaugural, I said: "The power confided to me will be used to hold, occupy, and possess the

property and places belonging to the government, and to collect the duties and imposts." This had your distinct approval at the time; and, taken in connection with the order I immediately gave General Scott, directing him to employ every means in his power to strengthen and hold the forts, comprises the exact domestic policy you now urge, with the single exception that it does not propose to abandon Fort Sumter.

Again, I do not perceive how the reinforcement of Fort Sumter would be done on a slavery or a party issue, while that of Fort Pickens would be on a more national and patriotic one.

The news received yesterday in regard to St. Domingo certainly brings a new item within the range of our foreign policy; but up to that time we have been preparing circulars and instructions to ministers and the like, all in perfect harmony, without even a suggestion that we had no foreign policy.

Upon your closing propositions—that "whatever policy we adopt, there must be an energetic prosecution of it.

> "For this purpose it must be somebody's business to pursue and direct it incessantly.
>
> "Either the President must do it himself, and be all the while active in it, or
>
> "Devolve it on some member of his cabinet. Once adopted, debates on it must end, and all agree and abide"—I remark that if this must be done, I must do it. When a general line of policy is adopted, I apprehend there is no danger of its being changed without good reason, or continuing to be a subject of unnecessary debate; still, upon points arising in its progress I wish, and suppose I am entitled to have, the advice of all the cabinet.
>
> Your obedient servant,
>
> A. Lincoln.[21]

Lincoln's written reply contains some dissembling,[22] but it seems clear that he did not deliver the document to Seward.[23] Most historians tend to believe he delivered some variant to the Seward orally.[24] Regardless of what Lincoln actually did, two things *are* clear: Seward's April 1 memorandum (1) did not change

Lincoln's decision to resupply Fort Sumter, and (2) did not change Seward's relationship with the president.[25]

Indeed, the first line of Lincoln's April 1 reply references "[s]ince parting with you." This undoubtedly refers to a meeting that day with Seward and a Navy officer (David Porter) regarding details of the secret expedition to resupply Fort Pickens that was proceeding in parallel to Fort Sumter (but not under that aegis of the Navy Department—rather under Seward and the State Department).[26]

Besides his memorandum (and the Fort Pickens expedition), Seward on April 1 also urged the president to meet with a leading Virginia Unionist, George Summers. That led to a same-day telegram by Seward to the man spearheading the fight against secession in that state: "The president desires your attendance at Washington as soon as convenient." After some confusion about the telegram, Summers, who needed to stay in Richmond to ensure that the Virginia convention's secession vote on April 4 would come out the right way, sent fellow-Unionist, John Baldwin; Baldwin had a one-on-one meeting with the president on April 4.[27]

Finally, on April 1, Justice John Campbell called on Seward to ask about the status of Fort Sumter, especially given what Ward Hill Lamon had told South Carolina Governor Francis Pickens. Disavowing Lamon's authority to speak for the president, Seward responded that Lincoln might resupply the fort, "but would not do so without notice to South Carolina's governor."[28] Campbell, not surprisingly, recognized that this was a different message than Seward's prior advice. After (purportedly) separately consulting with the president, Seward returned and handed Campbell a note (in Seward's handwriting): "I am satisfied the government will not undertake to supply Fort Sumter without giving notice to Governor Pickens." To explain this new message, Seward told Campbell that Lincoln's "ears are open to everyone, and they fill his head with schemes for its supply. I do not think that he will adopt any of them."[29]

On April 3, while the Cabinet was again meeting to discuss the fate of Fort Sumter (and the planning to resupply it continued to move forward in New York City), a small schooner showing an American flag was shelled as it attempted to enter Charleston's harbor.[30] That same day, Henry Raymond's *New York Times* (channeling Seward's April 1 memorandum) had a lead editorial: "Wanted—A Policy" (advocating a policy that would promote "a Union Party in every Southern State"); the next day Thurlow Weed's *Albany Evening Journal* followed suit, arguing that it would be a mistake for the federal government to "coerce" the secessionists and urging instead a policy of "reconciliation."[31] Besides giving Lincoln a headache, Seward's back-channel attempts in the press to change Lincoln's mind on Sumter proved as unavailing as his April 1 memorandum.

On April 4, the same day Lincoln was meeting with Virginia Unionist John Baldwin,[32] the Virginia convention (as George Summers had predicted) decisively voted against secession by a 90 to 45 margin. After the result, one Virginia Unionist delegate exclaimed: "That vote decided that Virginia would not commit the suicidal act of secession. The harpoon went into the vital spot of the whale, and . . . it will be but a little while before his white belly appears on the surface."[33] This good news did not alter Lincoln's thinking or decision-making as to resupplying Sumter, however; perhaps the margin only served to embolden the president—that he could resupply the fort with "food for hungry men" (a humanitarian mission), *and* keep Virginia in the Union (despite what every Union man below the Mason Dixon Line had been consistently telling both Seward and Lincoln).[34]

The Die Is Cast

On April 6, Robert Chew (a State Department clerk selected by Seward) was tasked by the president to deliver a message (ASAP) to South Carolina Governor

Francis Pickens.[35] Lincoln's message: that the governor should "expect an attempt will be made to supply Fort Sumter with provisions only."[36]

On April 7, as rumors were flying around Washington about what the federal government was (or was not) planning to do, Justice Campbell (prompted by the Confederate commissioners) asked Seward about Fort Sumter. Seward sent back a cryptic note: "Faith as to Sumter fully kept. Wait and see."[37] Unsatisfied, the commissioners that night went to Seward's house demanding a response to their month-old letter requesting a formal audience. The next day they received the response (which Seward had prepared in March): the United States would not recognize the Confederacy, nor would the Secretary of State be "at liberty to hold official intercourse with them."[38]

The commissioners swiftly replied with "a sharp and caustic letter," stating that Seward was "persistently wedded to those fatal theories of construction of the Federal Constitution, always rejected by the statesmen of the South"; predicting "blood and mourning," their letter concluded: "the undersigned, in behalf of their Government and people, accept the gage of battle thus thrown to them."[39] An even more enraged Campbell (since he had dealt with Seward face to face) sent a separate letter, accusing him of "systematic duplicity."[40]

On the same day the commissioners and Campbell were unloading their fury on Seward (April 8), Chew arrived in Charleston and delivered Lincoln's message to Governor Pickens. This led to the military forces ringing the harbor being put on full alert.

The Confederate government in Montgomery, Alabama, now debated their options. Ultimately, with one dissent, Davis and his cabinet instructed General Pierre Beauregard in Charleston to demand immediate evacuation of the fort and, if refused, to begin an assault.[41] On April 12 at 4:30 a.m. (with no resupply by the Fox expedition in sight), shelling began;[42] a day and a half later, Major Robert Anderson surrendered the fort. The American Civil War had begun.

In Washington on April 14 the Cabinet met to consider what to do in response to the attack on (and surrender of) Fort Sumter.[43] One (critical) thing that informed its deliberations was that, not unlike Pearl Harbor, the North had reacted overwhelmingly in outrage at the "first shot" and patriotically vowed allegiance to support the Union cause.[44] After the president and his Cabinet reached a compromise agreement on how many men to call into service (75,000 for 90 days), Lincoln pondered whether to call Congress into an immediate session to consider wartime legislation. Seward's advice was "no": alluding to Charles I, he told the president that "history tells us that kings who call extra parliaments lose their heads."[45] Based on that sage advice, Lincoln decided he would wait and call Congress into session on the Fourth of July.[46]

Lincoln's call for 75,000 troops was met with great enthusiasm in the North. But in the Border States it was that call to arms—not the Fort Sumter attack and surrender—that routed all traces of Union sentiment previously in evidence (and growing).[47] On April 17, the Virginia convention voted 88 to 55 for secession; and in May, Arkansas, North Carolina, and Tennessee joined Virginia.[48] Four years later, and with over 700,000 people killed (2 percent of the American population), the Civil War would end.

Notes

1. This chapter's title comes from Lincoln's second Inaugural Address on March 4, 1865, in which he felt it prudent to use the passive voice: "Both parties depricated war, but one of them would *make* war rather than let the nation survive, and the other would *accept* war rather than let it perish. And the war came." (Roy Basler (ed.), *The Collected Works of Abraham Lincoln,* Volume 8, p. 972 Rutgers University Press 1953-55).

2. Both Weed and Raymond were in accord with what Seward wrote in his famous/infamous "Some Thoughts for the President's Consideration" memorandum. And they thought the

president would be "in accord" with its contents. They planned to publish both Seward's memorandum and the president's reply in the *Albany Evening Journal* (Weed's newspaper) and the *New York Times* (Raymond's newspaper), along with "a vigorous editorial endorsement of the program." Walter Stahr, *Seward: Lincoln's Indispensable Man*, pp. 270-71 (Simon & Schuster 2012). When that did not go according to the plan, the two men had to go to Plan B (see infra note 31 (and accompanying text)).

3. Stahr, supra note 2, p. 271. David Potter termed the document as Seward being "at the end of his tether," his "last writhing paroxym in the struggle against circumstance," "mere blind gambling," "slap-dash improvision," and "baseless phantasy." David Potter, *Lincoln and His Party in the Secession Crisis*, pp. 370-71 (Louisiana State University Press 1995 (originally Yale University Press 1942)). Frederick Bancroft termed it "a gorgeous and dangerous scheme," the "reckless invention of a mind driven to desperate extremes, as the sole means of escape from ruin." *The Life of William H. Seward*, Volume 2, pp. 134-35 (Harper & Row 1900). Michael Burlingame is of the view that Seward was "frantic" and acting "rashly"; he termed the document: "Seward's offer to take over the Administration"; and he later called it "haughty" and "bizarre." Michael Burlingame, *Abraham Lincoln: A Life*, Volume II, pp. 117-19 (Johns Hopkins University Press 2009). British historian Nigel Hamilton (biographer of British World War II General Bernard Montgomery) has most recently weighed in, calling Seward's memorandum an attempted "coup d'etat." *Lincoln vs. Davis: The War of the Presidents*, pp. 128-34, 582-83 (Little, Brown and Company 2024). Even Seward's most recent biographer, Walter Stahr, wrote that "[t]he usual interpretation of Seward's memorandum is that Seward was *insane* to seek a foreign war and *insane*

to think Lincoln would yield control of the administration." supra note 2, p. 272 (emphasis added).

4. Seward April 1, 1981, Memorandum to Lincoln (Lincoln Papers, Library of Congress); Frederick W. Seward, *Seward at Washington: 1846-61*, p. 535 (Derby and Miller 1891); John M. Taylor, *William Henry Seward: Lincoln's Right Hand*, Appendix, pp. 308-09 (HarperCollins 1991). See also Potter, *Lincoln and His Party*, supra note 3, pp. 368-39; Daniel Crofts, *Reluctant Confederates: Upper South Unionists in the Secession Crisis*, pp. 298-300 (University of North Carolina Press 1987). Seward's son Frederick hand-delivered a version—re-written by Frederick (to ensure readability)—directly to Lincoln; Frederick Seward, *Reminiscence of a War-Time Statesman and Diplomat, 1830-1915*, pp. 149-50 (G.P. Putnam's Sons 1916); Stahr, supra note 2, p. 270.

5. See supra note 3.

6. Daniel Crofts, "Secession Winter: William Henry Seward and the Decision for War," *New York History*, pp. 252-53 (July 1984) & *Reluctant Confederates*, supra note 4, pp. 298-300; Patrick Sowle, "A Reappraisal of Seward's Memorandum of 1861, to Lincoln," *Journal of Southern History* 1967; Kinley Braver, "Seward's 'Foreign War Panacea': An Interpretation," *New York History* (1974). See also Lawrence Denton, *William Henry Seward and the Secession Crisis*, pp. 140-44 (McFarland & Company 2009); Stahr, supra note 2, pp. 269-72.

Interestingly, it was Daniel Potter who wrote: "The supreme task of the historian, and one of the most superlative difficulty, is to see the past through the imperfect eyes of those who lived it." *The South and the Sectional Conflict*, pp. 245-46 (Louisiana State University Press 1968). See also "The Critical Signpost on the Journey Toward Secession" in Michael Cooper's *Approaching Civil War and Southern History*, p. 134 (Louisiana State University Press 2019) (with respect to historians' praise of Lincoln's rejection of any territorial compromise, "that interpretation comes at the study of history backward, with hindsight as headlights. No one in the crisis of 1860-61, not even Lincoln, could read the future.").

7. David Donald, *Lincoln*, p. 289 (Simon & Schuster 1996); Burlingame, supra note 3, Volume II, pp. 108-09.

8. Both the *Norfolk Times* (March 21, 1861) and the *New York Tribune* (March 27, 1861) termed the administration's policy as "masterly inactivity" [harkening back to Lincoln's post-election silence]. Potter, *Lincoln and His Party*, supra note 3, pp. 329-31. On the other hand, the *New York Herald* (April 7, 1861) called the administration "imbecile and weak." And the *Washington States and Union* (March 21, 1861) demanded that Lincoln "show his hand; we want him to let us know decidedly and unequivocally what he means to do.... The people are claiming for a policy." See also Burlingame, supra note 3, Volume II, pp. 103-04.

9. For example, David Davis (Lincoln's close friend and campaign manager at the 1860 Convention—and later his nominee to the U.S. Supreme Court) acknowledged that the president "lacks will" and "yields to pressure." Henry Davis March 21, 1861, Letter to Samuel DuPont (DuPont Papers, Hagley Museum, Wilmington, Delaware); see also Burlingame, supra note 3, Volume II, p. 103. On March 28, 1861, Charles Francis Adams wrote in his diary: "the course of the President is drifting the country into war, by its want of decision.... For my part I see nothing but incompetency in the head. The man is not equal to the hour." (quoted in Glyndon Van Deusen, *William Henry Seward*, p. 281 (Oxford University Press 1967). Even Lord Richard Lyons, the British Minister, had reported to the Home Office: "[Lincoln has not demonstrated] any natural talents to compensate for his ignorance of everything but Illinois village

politics." Lyons April 9, 1861, Letter to Russell (quoted in James Randall & Richard Current, *Lincoln the President: Last Full Measure*, p. 81 (Dodd, Mead & Co. 1945)).

10. See Chapter VI, note 23 (and accompanying text); Denton, supra note 6, p. 142. Even David Potter conceded that this part of Seward's memorandum was "nothing but a ... repetition of ideas ... he had expressed before." *Lincoln and His Party*, supra note 3, p. 368.

11. See Chapter VIII, note 45 (and accompanying text).

12. In fact, Fort Pickens stayed unmolested as the property of the United States for the duration of the Civil War. Burlingame, supra note 3, Volume II, p. 123; Taylor, supra note 4, p. 198.

13. Richard Current, *Lincoln and the First Shot*, p. 90 (Harper & Row 1963). As Daniel Crofts has explained, evacuating Sumter would "show Southern Unionists that federal policy was designed neither to benefit the Republican party nor to interfere with slavery." "Secession Winter," supra note 6, p. 253. Lincoln, moreover, knew that many Republican die-hards were already disposed to accept the evacuation of Fort Sumter as a military necessity, while unalterably opposed to abandoning Fort Pickens (indeed, one Ohio Republican wrote to Lincoln that he would go down in history with Benedict Arnold if he gave up the Florida fort). Burlingame, supra note 3, Volume II, pp. 109-10.

14. As we would learn later, the French did in fact interject themselves into Mexican affairs during the Civil War. Stahr, supra note 2, pp. 326-27, 440-46; James McPherson, *Battle Cry of Freedom: The Civil War Era*, pp. 553-54, 683-84 (Oxford University Press 1988); see also William Hardy, "South of the Border: Ulysses S. Grant and the French Intervention," *Civil War History* (2008).

There were additional reports of France and England trying to "pick up any little advantages that may offer themselves" as a result of the constitutional crisis. Stahr, supra note 2, p. 271; Denton, supra note 6, p. 144. See also Frederick Seward, *Reminiscences,* supra note 4, pp. 148-49 (Seward was concerned that "[t]he 'Monroe Doctrine' could be safely ignored, and the interference of America need not be feared.").

15. The importance of foreign recognition was very much on Seward's mind at this time. See supra Chapter VIII, note 42 (and accompanying text); see also Burlingame, supra note 3, Volume II, p. 118.

16. See Chapter V, note 27 (and accompanying text). See also Burlingame, supra note 3, Volume II, p. 118.

17. Crofts, "Secession Winter," supra note 6, p. 252 & *Reluctant Confederates,* supra note 4, p. 299.

18. See, e.g., Burlingame, supra note 3, Volume II, p. 118.

19. Braver, supra note 6, pp. 152-56 (Seward wanted "the maintenance of peace both at home and abroad."); Sowle, supra note 6, pp. 234-45; Crofts, "Secession Winter," supra note 6, p. 253 & *Reluctant Confederates,* supra note 4, pp. 299-300.

20. See supra note 3. And, in fact, Seward did send messages to the foreign ministers of Spain, France, and England regarding San Domingo and Mexico. Stahr, supra note 2, pp. 274-75; F. Seward, supra note 4, pp. 540-43.

21. Basler, supra note 1, Volume 4, p. 317. As David Donald noted, other than this document "Lincoln left no record of how he felt about [Seward's] extraordinary document. *Lincoln,* supra note 7, p. 290.

22. For example, regarding the policy set forth in the Inaugural Address, both Lincoln and Seward knew that the Cabinet had been vacillating on resupplying or evacuating Fort Sumter since the inauguration. Moreover, as noted above, Lincoln had himself

de-coupled Sumter from Pickens, and understood the domestic political implication of that de-coupling.

23. There is no copy in Seward's papers. Frederick Seward undoubtedly felt he had to reference it since his treatise on his father (as well as his own memoir) came out after Nicolay and Hay's multi-volume biography on Lincoln had revealed the April 1 memorandum (and Lincoln's written reply) for the first time. Frederick's commentary on the president's reply is merely that it was "kind and dignified," also noting that before the month was over the question had in fact changed from slavery to union. F. Seward, supra note 4, pp. 535-36 and Frederick Seward, *Reminiscences,* supra note 4, pp. 149-50.

24. Donald, *Lincoln,* supra note 7, p. 290; Stahr, supra note 2, pp. 272-73; Taylor, supra note 4, p. 151. It is also possible that Lincoln said nothing. Almost exactly 100 years later, a just-inaugurated vice president, Lyndon Johnson, sent an even more audacious document to the new president, John Kennedy, seeking his approval of an executive order granting the vice president "general supervision" over numerous government agencies, and directing that Cabinet secretaries and department chiefs give LBJ copies of all important documents sent to the president. JFK decided to simply ignore the memorandum; some of his aides, however, leaked it to the press (comparing it to Seward's April 1 memorandum). Robert Caro, *The Years of Lyndon Johnson: The Passage of Power*, pp. 169-72 (Alfred Knopf 2012); Robert Dallek, *Flawed Giant: Lyndon Johnson and His Times, 1961-1973*, pp. 8-9 (Oxford University Press 1998); Jeff Shesol, *Mutual Contempt: Lyndon Johnson, Robert Kennedy, and the Feud That Defined a Decade*, pp. 64-65 (W.W. Norton 1992). Rebuffed by Kennedy's silence, Johnson did not press the issue; later he conceded to his protégé, Bobby Baker ("Little Lyndon"—Secretary of the U.S.

Senate): "If I learned anything last year, it's that Jack Kennedy's a lot tougher, and maybe a lot smarter, than I thought he was." Shesol, supra this note, p. 66.

25. C. Evan Stewart, *Law in American History (And in Mine)* (Chapter XXVII) (Twelve Tables Press 2025). Stahr, supra note 2, p. 273; Taylor, supra note 4, p. 151. As David Donald noted: perhaps one reason for Lincoln's restrained reaction to Seward's memorandum was that "it contained a considerable measure of truth." *"We Are Lincoln Men": Abraham Lincoln and the Friends*, pp. 152-53 (Simon & Schuster 2003); see also Norman Ferrisi, "Lincoln and Seward in Civil War Diplomacy: Their Relationship at the Outset Reexamined," *Journal of the Abraham Lincoln Association* (1991).

26. Secretary of the Navy Gideon Welles did not learn of the Pickens expedition until April 5 (the reason for secrecy was fear of Southern holdovers in the Navy Department). There is a big historical brouhaha about whether the assignment of the vessel *Powhattan* to the Pickens expedition was an attempt by Seward to "sabotage" the Sumter relief effort. Welles disliked Seward immensely and was very jealous of Seward's influence with the president. Just before Seward's death (when no reply could be made because of Seward's poor health), Welles launched various public broadsides against Seward, including the *Powhattan* "sabotage." Burlingame gives full credence to this story (supra note 3, Volume II, pp. 111-17), as does (not surprisingly) Nigel Hamilton, *Lincoln vs. Davis: The War of the Presidents*, pp. 137-42 (Little, Brown and Company 2024). For a more measured (and balanced) account, see Stahr, supra note 2, pp. 273-74, 276-78; Crofts, *Reluctant Confederates*, supra note 4, p. 439, n.47. See also Donald, *Lincoln*, supra note 7, pp. 290-92; Taylor, supra note 4, pp. 156-57; Denton, supra note 6, pp. 153-54. In any event, and as James McPherson noted: "In the end this [brouhaha] made

no difference to the outcome of the successful reinforcement of Pickens or the failure at Fort Sumter." *Tried by War: Abraham Lincoln as Commander in Chief*, pp. 19-20 (Penguin Press 2008).

27. There is "considerable" debate among historians as to whether Lincoln pledged to Baldwin on April 4 that he would evacuate Fort Sumter if Virginia were to terminate the secession convention. Compare Stahr, supra note 2, pp. 275-76 (doubtful) with Burlingame, supra note 3, Volume II, pp. 119-23 (yes) with Current, *Lincoln and the First Shot*, supra note 13, p. 95 ("Lincoln thought he had made it clear ... [in a conversation that] became more and more unpleasant, more and more confused.") with Crofts, *Reluctant Confederates*, supra note 4, pp. 301-06 and Denton, supra note 6, pp. 147-48 (there are conflicting accounts—"no conclusive answer is possible").

One thing seems clear out of the disparate versions of Lincoln's interactions with the Southern Unionists at this time: the president was more skeptical than was Seward as to their true loyalty to the Union. As Lincoln remarked to one Virginia visitor: "Yes! your Virginia people are good Unionists, but it is always with an *if*!" Current, *Lincoln and the First Shot*, supra note 13, p. 96 (the Southern Unionists were "white crows"—"a contradiction in terms"); Taylor, supra note 4, p. 159.

Whatever was said during this meeting the process for resupplying Fort Sumter continued without delay—and Lincoln made his "go" decision on that day. See infra note 34 (and accompanying text).

28. Stahr, supra note 2, p. 274; Taylor, supra note 4, p. 155; Potter, *Lincoln and His Party*, supra note 3, pp. 347-48; Burlingame, supra note 3, Volume II, p. 113. See also Campbell April 3, 1861, letter to Davis, *The Papers of Jefferson Davis*, Volume 7, pp. 88-89 (Haskell Monroe et al., eds.) (Louisiana State University Press 1971-2003).

29. Whether Seward was purposefully deceiving Campbell or continued to believe he (somehow) could yet change the president's mind on Sumter is unclear. Burlingame, supra note 3, Volume II, p. 113. It is indisputable, however, that Seward was continuing to facilitate Southern Unionists meeting with Lincoln as late as April 13. Denton, supra note 6, p. 158.

30. Burlingame, supra note 3, Volume II, p. 124.

31. Crofts, *Reluctant Confederates,* supra note 4, pp. 301-02; Burlingame, supra note 3, Volume II, p. 119; Denton, supra note 6, p. 145. These editorials were the Plan B after the initial plan for Seward's April 1 memorandum did not pan out. See supra note 2 (and accompanying text).

32. See supra note 27 (and accompanying text).

33. Crofts, *Reluctant Confederates,* supra note 4, pp. 308-10; Burlingame, supra note 3, Volume II, p. 120 (reporting a 89-45 vote).

34. McPherson, *Tried by War,* supra note 26, pp. 20-21. His April 5 and April 7 meetings with Virginia Unionists would have certainly disabused Lincoln of any such notion. Crofts, *Reluctant Confederates,* supra note 4, pp. 301-06; Denton, supra note 6, pp. 148-49.

These meetings were, in fact, academic insofar as the president had already told Fox on April 4 that he had decided "to let the [Sumter] expedition go." F. Seward, p. 536. Lincoln also notified Major Anderson on April 4 that a resupply force was on its way. Crofts, *Reluctant Confederates,* supra note 4, p. 440 n.48; Burlingame, supra note 3, Volume II, pp. 122-23; Taylor, supra note 4, p. 155.

One of Baldwin's fellow Virginia Unionists, Samuel Price, vividly remembered Baldwin telling him that Lincoln said on April 4: "I wish you had come sooner":

> When this remark of his was repeated to me, I remember that it chilled the very blood in my veins. I was, as you know, an intense Union man, and thought I saw that unless the Union party was upheld by the National Administration, that Virginia would inevitably take position with her Southern sisters; and I inferred from this remark of Mr. Lincoln, that he had taken a step, which he could not retrace, inconsistent with the view we were urging upon him, and which would result in war and bloodshed.

As Daniel Crofts concluded: "The abortive Baldwin interview was indeed 'too late.' So failed the last card Seward had to play in trying to change Lincoln's mind about Sumter." *Reluctant Confederates,* supra note 4, p. 306. See also Current, *Lincoln and the First Shot,* supra note 13, p. 112 (Current believed Lincoln said "It is too late now" to Virginia Unionist John Botts on April 7.); Denton, supra note 6, p. 155. Whether Lincoln made the "too late" comment to Baldwin on April 4 or to Botts on April 7 (or to both) will remain—just as whether the president suggested/promised a fort for Virginia trade to either man—an unresolved question(s) in history. Crofts, *Reluctant Confederates,* supra note 4, pp. 301-06; Denton, supra note 6, p. 149; William Harris, "The Southern Unionist Critique of the Civil War," *Civil War History* (1985). Lincoln's leading biographer believes that "[t]he evidence of [Lincoln's] proposed bargain with Virginia Unionists is murky, and any conclusion has to be tentative." Donald, *Lincoln,* supra note 7, pp. 290, 644; see also McPherson, *Tried by War,* supra note 26, p. 14 ("Whether Lincoln made such a proposal, and would have carried it out, must remain forever moot.").

35. As with many events of these momentous days, historians disagree about many key details as to who was present and knew of Lincoln's dispatching of Chew. See, e.g., Current, *Lincoln and the First Shot*, supra note 13, pp. 108-10; Stahr, supra note 2, p. 278; Burlingame, supra note 3, Volume II, pp. 123-24; Denton, supra note 6, p. 154.

36. Lincoln April 6, 1861, note to Chew (Basler, supra note 1, Volume 4, pp. 323-24). Earlier that same day, James Harvey, a Washington correspondent for two newspapers, sent a telegram to a prominent lawyer in South Carolina: "Positively determined not to withdraw Anderson. Supplies go immediately, supported by a naval force under Stringham, if their landing be resisted. A Friend." Critics of Seward have charged that he purposefully leaked the information to Harvey and thus was complicit in Harvey's "treason." Burlingame, supra note 3, Volume II, p. 116. There is good reason to doubt Seward's complicity, however, because (1) he knew Stringham was not in charge of the naval fleet, and (2) he was still bringing Southern Unionists to meet with the president to dissuade him from resupplying Fort Sumter; so leaking that information (especially to a prominent South Carolinian) would be nonsensical (i.e., to what end?). See Danial Crofts, "James E. Harvey and the Secession Crisis," *Pennsylvania Magazine of History and Biography* (April 1979). See also Stahr, supra note 2, p. 278; Denton, supra note 6, p. 154; Van Deusen, p. 285.

As with many Civil War issues, historians have long debated *when* Lincoln made an "irreversible" decision to resupply Fort Sumter. Lincoln retrospectively assigned April 6; as set forth above, March 29 (the Cabinet meeting) or April 4 (Lincoln's instructions to Fox and Anderson) have many supporters. See Donald, *Lincoln*, supra note 7, pp. 292, 644; Crofts, *Reluctant Confederates*, supra note 4, p. 440 note 48; Potter, *Lincoln and His Party*, supra note 3, pp. 362-63. Regardless, as Michael Burlingame has written, once Lincoln sent notice to Governor Pickens, the "die was finally cast." supra note 3, Volume II, p. 124.

As explained by James McPherson, Civil War historians have broken into three camps vis-à-vis Lincoln's motives and purposes for his resupply plan for Fort Sumter. The *first* is essentially political: that he believed only a war would sustain his administration and the Republican Party; thus, he deliberately manipulated the firing of the first shot on the fort. The *second* is that he feared that giving up Sumter would weaken the administration and correspondingly strengthen the Confederate government (especially in the eyes of foreign governments); hoping for peace, but willing to risk war, Lincoln gave Jefferson Davis the choice of peace or war. The *third* is that Lincoln would have been satisfied to maintain the status quo (peace), "but probably expected the Confederates to open fire; either way he won." McPherson finds "interpretation 3 … [the] most plausible." *Battle Cry of Freedom*, supra note 14, p. 272, n.78; see also McPherson, *Tried by War*, supra note 26, pp. 20-21 (terming Lincoln's ploy: "Heads I win; tails you [Jefferson Davis] lose").

David Donald also weighed in on this debate (*Lincoln*, supra note 7, pp. 292-93) and concluded:

> The area of disagreement in this controversy has perhaps been exaggerated: all authorities agree that Lincoln wished to avoid war and all agree that he was willing to run the risk of war rather than evacuate Fort Sumter. None of these able scholars has, in my opinion, given enough attention to Lincoln's newness in Washington, his inexperience as an administrator, and his fatigue

> after his exhausting journey and inauguration. Nor has Lincoln's essential passivity, his preference to react to events rather than take the initiative, been sufficiently stressed.

See also Richard Current, *Lincoln and the First Shot*, supra note 13; Richard Current, *Speaking of Abraham Lincoln: The Man and the Meaning for Our Times*, pp. 61-78 (University of Illinois Press 1983); *Why the Civil War Came*, pp. 5-30 (Gabor Boritt ed.) (Oxford University Press 1996); and infra, Epilogue, note 6.

Clearly Lincoln believed that his order to resupply Sumter could well trigger armed conflict, given his meeting on April 6 with the governors of Indiana, Maine, Illinois, Wisconsin, Michigan, and Ohio (all hard-liners), at which he expressly asked for military assistance "when the ball opened ... [with Washington] the first [city] that will be attacked." Burlingame, supra note 3, Volume II, p. 126.

This debate bears a striking resemblance to a similar debate among historians about President Franklin Roosevelt's motives in the fall of 1941, when he confronted the Empire of Japan with crippling sanctions. See Ted Morgan, *FDR: A Biography*, pp. 573-624 (Simon & Schuster 1985); Kenneth Davis, *FDR: The War President, 1940-43*, pp. 313-21, 333-38 (Random House 2000).

37. F. Seward, supra note 4, p. 538; Stahr, supra note 2, pp. 278-79; Burlingame, supra note 3, Volume II, p. 124. On April 6 (presumably triggered by Harvey's telegram of that same day—see supra note 36), Jefferson Davis wrote to Justice Campbell, expressing uncertainty whether the telegram was "sent here to deceive us," and concluding that he would await "the determination of a problem which it belongs to the Govt of the United States to control." *Jefferson*

Davis: The Essential Writings, pp. 208-09 (William Cooper ed.) (Random House 2003).

38. Seward's April 10, 1861, memorandum to the Department of State's official files regarding his reply to the commissioners is at F. Seward, supra note 4, p. 538.

39. F. Seward, supra note 4, p. 537.

40. John Campbell, "Facts of History," *Southern Historical Society Papers*, 38-41 (1917) (originally prepared December 20, 1873). Duplicitous or not, even David Potter concluded: "[A]t a heavy cost to his personal credit, Seward had prevented for four full weeks the precipitation of a diplomatic crisis which might have had immediate military repercussions." *Lincoln and His Party*, supra note 3, p. 349.

41. The Confederate government's deliberations are well set forth in Burlingame, supra note 3, Volume II, pp. 126-29. (Secretary of State Robert Toombs warned against striking the first blow: "You will wantonly strike a hornet's nest which ... now quiet, will swarm out and sting us to death."). See also William Davis, *Jefferson Davis: The Man and His Hour*, pp. 321-25 (HarperCollins 1991); *The Papers of Jefferson Davis*, Volume 7, pp. 88-104 (Haskell Monroe et al., eds.) (Louisiana State University Press 1991-2003).

42. See *The Diary of Edmund Ruffin*, Volume I, pp. 581-604 (William Scarborough ed.) (Louisiana State University Press 1972) (Ruffin, who fired the first shot, details the assault on Fort Sumter).

Also on April 12, the expedition to Fort Pickens arrived without incident. Denton, supra note 6, p. 157; Taylor, supra note 4, p. 158.

43. On that same day Charles Sumner was lamenting to the U.S. Attorney for Massachusetts: "We are now reaping the fruits of *Sewardism* throughout the winter—demoralizing our energies and planting distrust every where but no where more than in the Slave

States themselves. I have deplored that *policy of insincerity*, & my chief hope now is that it will be renounced." Sumner April 14, 1861, letter to R. Dana, *The Selected Correspondence of Charles Sumner*, Volume 2, p. 64 (Beverly Palmer ed.) (Northeastern University Press 1990).

44. McPherson, *Battle Cry of Freedom*, supra note 14, pp. 274-75 ("The people have gone stark mad."; "the change in pubic sentiment here [New York City] is wonderful—almost miraculous."; "It seems as if we were never alive till now; never had a country till now."); Current, *Lincoln and the First Shot*, supra note 13, pp. 159-61; Burlingame, supra note 3, Volume II, p. 138.

45. Stahr, supra note 2 p. 280.

46. One key outcome of this decision was that Lincoln used that period to exercise "extra" constitutional power to ensure that secession fever did not overwhelm Maryland. See C. Evan Stewart, *The Worst Supreme Court Decisions, Ever! (And Related Tales)* (Chapter XVII) (Twelve Tables Press 2024); Burlingame, supra note 3, Volume II, pp. 149-54.

47. James Randall & David Donald, *The Civil War and Reconstruction*, pp. 188-89 (D.C. Heath and Company 1961) (Lincoln's call for troops "served in one flash to alienate that whole mass of Union sentiment"). For an excellent, recent analysis of which Northerners enthusiastically responded to Lincoln's call to enlist, see Richard Edwards, "Saving the Republic, Sinking the Republicans: Unraveling the Anomalous 1862 Midterms and Their Consequences," *Civil War History* (September 2025). For a collection of excellent essays on Union sentiment in the South *after* the Civil War began, see *Enemies of the Country: New Perspectives on Unionists in the Civil War South* (John Inscoe & Robert Kenzer, eds.) (University of Georgia Press 2001).

48. Crofts, *Reluctant Confederates*, supra note 4, pp. 337-52; McPherson, *Battle Cry of Freedom*, supra note 14, pp. 278-84.

Even Unionist William Rives—with whom Lincoln had his famous colloquy regarding a trade of Virginia for Fort Sumter (see supra Chapter VII note 40 (and accompanying text))—voted for secession ("The Government being already overthrown by revolution, I vote 'aye.'") A revised, final vote for Virginia secession (with some changing their tallies and absentees weighing in) was 103 to 46. McPherson, *Battle Cry of Freedom*, supra note 14, p. 239 n.6.

Epilogue

Seward, in the view of most historians, was one of America's greatest Secretaries of State.[1] Not only did he keep the Confederacy from being recognized as an independent nation by England and France (a contrary result would have ended the Civil War—as a victory, but for the South), he wisely advised Lincoln on a multiplicity of matters both foreign and domestic over Lincoln's four years in office (1861-65).[2] Thus, for example, Seward counseled Lincoln on how to issue the emancipation proclamation from a position of strength versus weakness (advice that Lincoln acknowledged he had "entirely overlooked … [and that] struck [the president] with very great force.").[3] And once Seward made clear to Lincoln that he had no interest in succeeding the president, either in 1864 or in 1868, the two men moved to a greater level of personal intimacy. Their's was truly " a friendship that helped with the Civil War."[4]

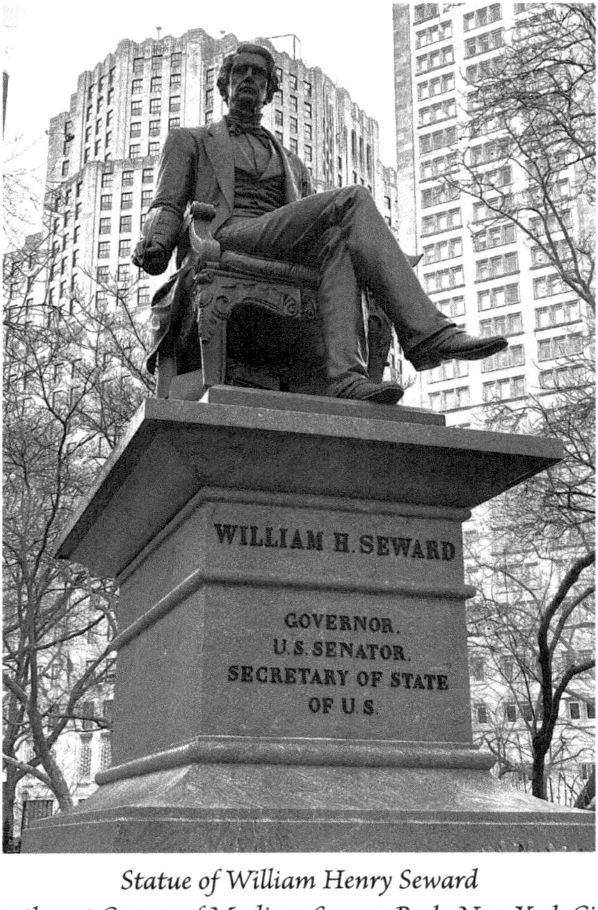

Statue of William Henry Seward
(Southwest Corner of Madison Square Park, New York City)
(Seward's head on Lincoln's body)
(author's collection)

So how should Seward's Southern Strategy during the Secession Winter be evaluated? It would not be historically accurate to conclude that it failed. Seward's strategy, in the post-election months, had indisputably bought the new administration time to get into place and start to wield the levers of power. After March 4, 1861, Seward's conciliatory policy, the dilatory dealings with the Southern commissioners, and his constant encouragement to Border States Unionists continued to work—witness the very strong anti-secession vote in Virginia on April 4. And although it appeared to Seward that Lincoln was (mostly) amenable to a conciliatory policy after March 4 in order to hold the Border States in the Union, the record seems clear that the president was never really on the same page with his Secretary of State.[5] Ultimately, it was Lincoln's decision whether to resupply Fort Sumter and risk a civil war.[6] What would have happened if Sumter had been evacuated and the May elections in Virginia taken place?[7] That is the stuff of counterfactual history.[8]

One thing Seward was *not* right about was his fear that taking up arms and forcibly trying to achieve reunion would divide the North.[9] Perhaps because of his ties to New York City's business leaders, who had strong commercial relationships with the South (especially with respect to cotton), Seward was not prepared for the patriotic unanimity that the firing on Fort Sumner spontaneously generated across the Northern States. But that unanimity was, in no small measure, based upon a belief that any conflict with the South would be quickly resolved in a decisive Northern victory.[10] Of course, that proved to be tragically wrong.[11]

But as to Seward's six-month struggle to keep the Border States in the Union (which he hoped would, at some point, bring about a peaceful reunion with the Cotton States), Henry Adams would later pose a question and then offer his own answer:

> [W]hat would have been the end of the matter if Mr. Seward had carried his point, and the conciliatory policy had become the policy of the Government[?] ... Like all such attempts at wisdom and moderation in times of heated passions and threatening war, it was swallowed up and crushed under the weight of brute force, that final tribunal to which human nature is subjected or subjects herself without appeal. Yet it is right to make the effort even if overruled.[12]

Notes

1. In addition to those treatises cited in Chapter I, note 1 regarding Seward's historical legacy as a great Secretary of State,

additional works to consult include: Robert Zoellick, *America in the World: A History of U. S. Diplomacy and Foreign Policy* (Twelve 2020); Joseph Fry, *Lincoln Seward, and U.S. Foreign Relations in the Civil War Era* (University Press of Kentucky 2019); Howard Jones, *Blue and Gray Diplomacy: A History of Union and Confederate Foreign Policy* (University of North Carolina Press 2010); Richard Immerman, *Empire for Liberty: A History of American Imperialism from Benjamin Franklin to Paul Wolfowitz* (Princeton University Press 2010); Philip Meyers, *Caution and Cooperation: The American Civil War in British-American Relations* (Kent State University Press 2008); Dean Mahin, *One War at a Time: The International Dimensions of the American Civil War* (Brassy's 1999); Ernest Paolino, *The Foundation of American Empire: William Henry Seward and U.S. Foreign Policy* (Cornell University Press 1973). See also Jay Sexton, "William H. Seward in the World," *The Journal of the Civil War Era* (2014); Michael Robinson, "William Henry Seward and the Onset of the Secession Crisis" *Civil War History* (2013).

2. Walter Stahr, *Seward: Lincoln's Indispensable Man*, pp. 290-92, 546-47 (Simon & Schuster 2012); James McPherson, *Battle Cry of Freedom: The Civil War Era*, pp. 388-91, 548-57 (Oxford University Press 1988); C. Evan Stewart, "Diplomat of the Civil War," *New York Archives* (Summer 2011). For an anti-Seward view(s) on this issue, see (not surprisingly) Michael Burlingame, *Abraham Lincoln: A Life*, Volume II, pp. 160-62 (Johns Hopkins University Press 2009); Nigel Hamilton, *Lincoln vs. Davis: The War of the Presidents*, pp. 123-42 (Little, Brown and Company 2024).

3. Stahr, supra note 2, pp. 342-43; McPherson, *Battle Cry of Freedom*, supra note 2, p. 505; Burlingame, supra note 2, Volume II, pp. 363-64.

4. David Donald, *"We Are Lincoln Men": Abraham Lincoln and His Friends*, pp. 146-76 (Simon & Schuster 2003); C. Evan Stewart, *Law in American History (And in Mine)* (Chapter XXVII) (Twelve Tables Press 2025).

After the Civil War began (and Lincoln became more comfortable exercising power in the midst of the constitutional crisis), Seward began to admire the president greatly. During this time he wrote to his wife: "Executive skill and vigor are rare qualities. The President is the best of us." Not leaving it here, however, Seward added that Lincoln needed "constant and assiduous cooperation." Seward June 5, 1861, letter to F. Seward (Frederick W. Seward, *Seward at Washington: 1846-61*, p. 590 (Derby and Miller 1891).

Right after Lincoln's re-election in 1864, Seward's evaluation was unconditional: "The election has placed our President beyond the pale of human envy or human harm, as he is above the pale of ambition. Henceforth all men will come to see him as … I have seen him—a true, loyal, patient, patriotic, and benevolent man." John M. Taylor, *William Henry Seward: Lincoln's Right Hand*, p. 234 (HarperCollins 1991). And after Lincoln's assassination (and the near fatal attempt on Seward's life that same night) in April 1865, Seward told a visitor (during his convalescence): "No knife was ever sharp enough to divide us upon any question of public policy, though we frequently arrived at the same conclusion through different processes of thought. Only once did we disagree in sentiment …: His 'colonization' scheme which I opposed on the self-evident principles all *natives* of a country have an *equal* right in its soil." Sebastian Page, "'A Knife Sharp Enough to Divide Us': William H. Seward, Abraham Lincoln, and Black Colonization," *Diplomatic History* (2016); see also Stahr, supra note 2, p. 341 (Seward: "I am always for bringing men and states *into* this Union, … never for taking any *out*.").

5. One leading Civil War historian has weighed in on "why" Abraham Lincoln (who considered the Great Compromiser, Henry Clay, his "beau ideal of a statesman") took a no-compromise approach throughout the Secession Winter; whereas William Henry Seward, theretofore the "radical" exponent of "A Higher Law" and an "irrepressible conflict," was the leading advocate of compromise during that same period. In his essay "Where Was Henry Clay? Lincoln and the Crisis of the Union" (pp. 139-53 in *Approaching Civil War and Southern History* (Louisiana State University Press 2019)), William Cooper identified three reasons for Lincoln's hard-line stance: "his ignorance of the South, his vigorous partisanship, and his visceral antislavery commitment." Id. p. 144.

As to the first, Cooper noted that Lincoln not only "knew so little about the South," he also had "no friends or even serious acquaintances among Southern politicians … [no one] who could educate him about the South and southern politics." As to the second, Cooper believed that Lincoln "acted like a partisan's partisan, not the leader of a country.… The evidence strongly suggests that he feared alienating his party's most fervent antislavery zealots." And as to the third, Cooper, after surveying Lincoln's public and private views on slavery, concluded that he had a deep and "visceral hatred of slavery"—it was morally "wrong." "Thus, for Lincoln, to accept any compromise that even theoretically permitted the possibility of expanding slavery meant turning from a vision he cherished both of past and future."

Cooper then contrasted these three Lincoln points with four for Seward. First, Seward "had a much better grasp than Lincoln of the political force of secession and the political reality facing the more moderate men in the … South." Second, Seward (and Weed) believed that expansion of slavery as a political issue had been resolved by the election of a Republican president in 1960. (See also supra Chapter IV, notes 8 and 10 (and accompanying text)). Third, Seward (and Weed) believed that if the Democratic Party reunited after 1860, it could well pose significant problems for the Republican Party, unless their party could grow beyond its 1860 base of support (39.8%); and the best way to broaden that party was to appeal to Unionists in the Upper South, focusing on the issue of Union (and *not* on sectional differences—e.g., slavery, slavery expansion). As for the anti-slavery, no-compromise wing of the Republican Party, Seward had advised Lincoln several times (see, e.g., Chapter VII, note 32 (and accompanying text)) that the (minority) wing of the party had nowhere else to go if the new administration became more conciliatory. [With respect to his third point, Cooper noted that there is "no evidence" that Lincoln was thinking about expanding the base of the Republican Party in 1860-61; of course, by 1864, the Republican Party did, in fact, become the Union Party. See Gary Gallagher, *The Union War*, p. 52 (Harvard University Press 2011); "Abraham Lincoln and the Politics of Union" in Michael Holt's *Political Parties and American Political Development from the Age of Jackson to the Age of Lincoln* (Louisiana State University Press 1992).]

Cooper's final Seward point is that Lincoln's hatred of slavery was "much deeper [and] more visceral." While "Seward did abhor slavery, [he never gave] it equal billing with freedom." (See also supra Chapter VII, note 32 (and accompanying text)). Seward "was willing to let [slavery] and the Southern political strength based on it become casualties of America's inevitable progress.... [A]fter the territorial issue had accomplished its political task in 1860, Seward was quite willing shelve it."

Cooper concluded that "despite his words, Lincoln in the great crisis of the Union did not look to Henry Clay.... Seward demonstrated himself, much more than Lincoln, a man of national outlook. In the winter of 1860-61 the New Yorker acted like the disciple of Clay. In this instance Seward had legitimate claim to the mantle of Henry Clay." Id. p. 153.

6. As discussed in Chapter IX, note 36 (and accompanying text), Lincoln's "real" reason for making his fateful decision is one of the most hotly debated, ongoing (and unresolvable) issues in historiography. James Randall (in McPherson's "2" camp) famously put it as follows:

> To say that Lincoln meant that the first shot would be fired by the other side *if a first shot was fired* is not to say that he maneuvered to have the first shot fired.

J.G. Randall, *Lincoln the President*, Volume 1, p. 350 (Dodd, Mead & Co. 1945-1955). As David Donald observed, Lincoln himself gave "several explanations of his course during the Sumter crisis." David Donald, *Lincoln*, p. 292-94 (Simon & Schuster 1996).

David Potter believed that Lincoln later second-guessed his decision:

> In the months that followed, Lincoln exhibited great forbearance and charity toward the south. That he did so may not be entirely a consequence of his personal magnanimity. It may also have derived from a conviction that, if the matter had been handled different—if, indeed, he had handled the matter differently—the conflict might have been averted.

David Potter, *Lincoln and His Party in the Secession Crisis*, p. 375 (Louisiana State University Press 1995).

7. Henry Adams later wrote that the Virginia elections were to be a "decisive point" in the efforts to avoid a civil war. Henry Adams, "The Great Secession Winter of 1860-61," *Proceedings of the Massachusetts Historical Society,* pp. 683-84 (1910).

8. For counterfactual histories on this score, see Daniel Crofts, *Reluctant Confederates: Upper South Unionists in the Secession Crisis,* pp. 353-55 (University of North Carolina Press 1987); Lawrence Denton, *William Henry Seward and the Secession Crisis* (McFarland & Company 2009), pp. 168-96.

9. Seward March 15, 1961, Memorandum to Lincoln (Lincoln Papers) (see supra Chapter VIII, note 19 (and accompanying text)); Crofts, *Reluctant Confederates,* supra note 8, pp. 357-58.

10. Southern Fire-Eaters thought exactly the same thing (except that *they* would be victorious, quickly). Frederick Seward, *Reminiscences of a War-Time Statesman and Diplomat, 1830-1915,* p. 153 (G.P. Putnam's Sons 1916); McPherson, *Battle Cry of Freedom,* supra note 2, pp. 269, 274-75, 309, 317; Burlingame, supra note 2, Volume II, p. 138; Richard Current, *Lincoln and the First Shot,* , p. 118 (Harper & Row 1963); Kenneth Stamp, *The Course of the Civil War,* pp. 140-45 (Prentice Hall 1965). Stephen Douglas issued a public statement on April 14 that "he was prepared to sustain the President in the exercise of all of his constitutional functions to preserve the Union." (*The Letters of Stephen Douglas,* pp. 509-10 (Robert Johannsen ed.) (University of Illinois Press 1961)); and even ex-president James Buchanan said: "The North will sustain the administration almost to a man." Winston Churchill, *The American Civil War,* p. 38 (Fairfax Press 1985).

11. Not surprisingly, as the North suffered major setbacks on the battlefield and a quick and easy victory proved illusory, the unanimity of Northern sentiment for the war dropped precipitously,

with partisan politics returning to pre-war levels and the Republican Party suffering significant losses in the 1862 elections. See Joel Silbey, *A Respectable Minority: The Democratic Party in the Civil War Era, 1860-1868*, p. 144 (Norton 1977); Adam Smith, *No Party Now: Politics in the Civil War North*, pp. 57-63 (Oxford University Press 2006). The months of July and August 1864 were the nadir of Northern enthusiasm for the war, with (in the words of Thurlow Weed) "Lincoln's re-election an impossibility.... The people are wild for peace." McPherson, *Battle Cry of Freedom*, supra note 2, pp. 760-61. The pressures on Lincoln at this point made his "life a hell," and on August 23 he composed his famous "blind memorandum," which he had his Cabinet secretaries endorse on the back sight unseen ("This morning, as for some days past, it seems exceedingly probable that this Administration will not be re-elected. Then it will be my duty to co-operate with the President elect, as to save the Union between the election and the inauguration; as he will have secured his election on such ground that he can not possibly save it afterwards."). Id. pp. 770-71; *The Collected Works of Abraham Lincoln*, Volume 7, p. 514 (Roy Basler ed.) (Rutgers University Press 1953-55). But with Sherman taking Atlanta on September 1 ("Atlanta is ours, and fairly won") and Sheridan's dramatic victories later that month in the Shenandoah Valley, the tide of the war—and Northern opinion—seemed to turn on a dime. McPherson, *Battle Cry of Freedom*, supra note 2, pp. 774-81. On election day (November 8), the Union Party (formerly the Republican Party) cruised to an easy victory in both the popular vote and the Electoral College. See Smith, supra this note, pp. 150-52 n.179. From that point on, the North was "in earnest ... to fight to the last." McPherson, *Battle Cry of Freedom*, supra note 2, p. 806.

12. Adams, supra note 7, pp. 683-84.

THE POWER OF ENZYMES

Your Ticket to a Healthier Life

THE POWER OF ENZYMES

Your Ticket to a Healthier Life

PAUL NEMIROFF, PhD, MD, FACS
with ARNOLD MANN

SORA LLC
PUBLISHING
Forsyth, Missouri

Published by Sora Publishing, LLC
15366 US Highway 160
Forsyth, MO 65653 USA

Mention of certain references in this book are historical information and do not suggest endorsement by the author or publisher. Internet addresses for resources provided in this book were accurate at the time the book went to press.

Cover design and layout: Jessica R. Koman
Editorial services: Meredith H. Pond
Photo of Dr. Paul Nemiroff: Becky Thurner
Photo of Arnold Mann: Linda Jane

Library of Congress Cataloging-in-Publication Data
Nemiroff, Paul M.
The Power of Enzymes: Your Ticket to a Healthier Life.
Includes glossary of enzymes, references, and index.
1. Enzymes—history, research, and therapeutic use.
2. Nutrition.
Mann, Arnold.

ISBN 978-0-9908919-0-1 (softcover edition)
ISBN 978-0-9908919-1-8 (e-book edition)

GENERAL DISCLAIMER
Information in this book is for educational purposes only. The author and the publisher assume no liability or responsibility for any adverse effects or consequences resulting from the suggestions, preparations, or procedures mentioned in this book. You must discuss all your medical issues with your health care professional. If you are currently under a health professional's care, you should share any major changes in your health immediately. Because this is a book (and not a medical consultation), please keep in mind that the information presented in this book may not apply to your case. In view of individual medical requirements, new research, and government regulations, it is the responsibility of you, the reader, to talk with your health care professional, before beginning any supplement or treatment program.

First Edition—Printed in the United States

TABLE OF CONTENTS

DEDICATION

To the memory of Dr. Edward Howell,

Father of Food Enzymes

INTRODUCTION

Discoveries that change human thinking are rare. Those that change thinking in the medical world, and our understanding of human health, are even more rare.

In 1924, a young physician by the name of Edward Howell was working his first job at the Lindlahr Sanitarium outside of Chicago when he made such a discovery, one which has given birth to an entirely new way of looking at human nutrition and health—through the power of enzymes.

The fascinating story told in this book takes us back to the beginning of mankind, when "food enzymes" contained in everything we ate assisted us in the digestion of these foods. That's the way Nature had set things up—with every living herbivore and carnivore achieving complete

digestion and full-body nutrition with the assistance of the living enzymes contained in the foods we consumed.

Things have changed over the past several hundred thousand years though, since early humans began cooking food. With cooking has come the reduction of enzymes and enzyme activity in most of the foods that make up our diet.

Our story begins with Dr. Howell trying to figure out why the daily doses of orange juice and fresh butter rubs are suddenly no longer having their beneficial effects on the gastrointestinal and skin problems plaguing the patients at the Lindlahr Sanitarium. The young physician is completely in the dark on this one, until a nurse mentions the word "pasteurization."

It was at that moment that Dr. Edward Howell's life work began.

We follow Howell's learning curve, starting with a close-up look at what an enzyme is. Howell called them "Nature's workers"—appropriately so, because enzymes are, without exaggeration, responsible for initiating and orchestrating virtually every aspect of life on this planet. How? The book takes us through the process step by step.

We learn about the food enzyme stomach, which exists throughout the animal kingdom in one form or another, including in humans.

With the advent of cooking, pasteurization, food processing and extended shelf life technologies, we learn what has happened to our food quality and our ability to digest food. The price we may be paying is incomplete digestion and impaired nutrition. Some scientists believe that partially digested foods may lead to inflammation. We also learn that inflammation appears to be the root of all evil when it comes to chronic diseases.

We see incomplete digestion in action. From local inflammation to the body-wide inflammatory cascade that is believed by many of today's scientists to breed chronic diseases, such as arthritis, heart disease, and even possibly cancer. We see how the introduction of food enzymes into our daily diet may improve our health.

And finally, we see how digestive enzyme supplements may bring Nature's "life element" back into our lives.

It's a fascinating story of science, intuition, and positive results. A story that can help us all lead healthier, perhaps even longer lives, through the power of enzymes.

So enjoy the journey.

Paul M. Nemiroff, PhD, MD, FACS

2014

A PERSONAL NOTE

By Anthony Collier

The first time I met Doc Howell was in November of 1977 at the Ft. Meyers Airport in Florida.

I was a 27-year-old graduate student, winding up my masters degree in business at DePaul University, and I had just taken a job at the National Enzyme Company (NEC) in Chicago, which he had founded back in 1932. Forty-five years later, the company was still a small mail-order operation run by the husband-wife team who bought it from Howell in 1955, freeing him up from the commercial aspects of enzymes so he could remain the pure scientist.

I was ambitious and full of ideas. I had plans for the company. So I had flown down to Florida to meet the

man who was the vision behind the business and learn what I could from him. And, to give him a chance to check me out. I did not realize that the education at the hands of my octogenarian mentor would involve some 50 trips to Florida spanning the next 12 years, and that this man's life mission would become my mission and give my life meaning I could never have imagined.

This was, after all, Dr. Edward Howell, the Father of Food Enzymes.

He was at the airport when I arrived. He was a slight gentleman, the son of German immigrants. Casually dressed, in light colors, he had a full head of silver hair. He was a small man with a large presence. His lively eyes knew me instantly. If only he could remember where he had left his car.

He was retired, and yet he was not.

"We've got a lot to do today," he said when he picked me up bright and early the next morning at my hotel and drove me to his home in north Ft. Myers. It was there that I got my first real glimpse of the man whose entire life had been devoted to the study of enzymes, culminating in two seminal books.

In the garage were dozens of 55-gallon steel drums, filled with the fruits of his research over the years. Parked

outside the small house was a Volkswagen bus, equipped with a cot and a small desk, which he used for monthly trips to the medical libraries in Tampa and Miami, where he would spend a week going through the latest research. He'd open and close the library every day, then go back to his van and type up his notes. At the end of the week he'd bring it all back home and spend the next three weeks putting it together.

He had been and always would be 100 percent German scientist.

But that first trip was devoted to me.

The first day he went through the ABCs of enzymes—how enzymes are contained in all our foods when they're fresh and raw and how our bodies use these food enzymes to digest these foods: proteases and lipases in meats; amylases in high carbohydrate foods, potatoes, fruits and vegetables; cellulases in high-fiber fruits and vegetables.

Then he got into the effects of heat on enzymes. A little bit of warming doesn't necessarily do any damage, "but if the water is warm enough to burn your finger, you're killing enzymes," he said.

The damage, he said, starts at about 108 degrees. Pasteurizing is done at either 165 degrees for 20 minutes or 188 degrees for 10 minutes. That kills about 90 percent

of enzymes. If you boil something at 212 degrees for a minute and a half, he said, you've pretty much killed all the enzymes in it. He went into sautéing, frying, baking and microwaving. He covered everything, from freezing to baking at 450 degrees.

He pulled studies demonstrating to me the importance of enzymes and that the human body was not meant to subsist on an enzyme-deficient diet. It was not natural. It didn't take long for me to realize that Dr. Howell was the supreme authority on food enzymes and that he was a brilliant man, completely devoted.

His devotion extended to his own eating habits, of course, which consisted of liberal helpings of uncooked fresh fruits and vegetables from his own "Enzyme Garden," which he fertilized with enzyme-rich fish entrails.

When we dined out, the word to the waiter was always, "Don't cook the veggies."

And of course he took his supplements before and after each meal.

He asked about my plans for the company, told me about his mission, and I made him a promise that I would do my best to fulfill that mission. He wanted the general public and the medical field to be made aware of the

health and therapeutic benefits of supplemental enzymes.

The bottom line: we clicked. He approved of me, and I had found a mentor.

Every three months I would fly down on a Thursday and spend a long weekend with him. Our days started at 9 a.m. sharp and ran 10 to 12 hours. He'd have everything ready—a four-inch-high stack of scientific papers—and he would take me through that week's learning curve.

One day I showed up 10 minutes late. He was pacing out front when I drove up.

"Why are you late?" he asked.

I told him breakfast was late.

"You don't have time to eat when you're here," he shot back. "This is too important."

He was dead serious. I grew to love the old man.

My lessons continued.

We spent an entire visit on the food enzyme stomach—the upper half of the human stomach where food enzymes do their work, pre-digesting up to 60 percent of what we eat, taking a lot of the burden off the overworked pancreas, and the immune system, which is often recruited to do digestive duties.

How important are food enzymes?

The evidence for this, Howell said, lies in the fact that human saliva is loaded with salivary amylase. Not so with other animals, except the dog that eats cooked food along with its human masters. But if you feed a dog raw food, within three weeks its saliva will be devoid of amylase, because it's no longer needed.

Howell did the study himself.

My quarterly lessons continued for 12 years, until 1988, two months before his death from pneumonia, at the age of 89.

I have done everything I can to keep the promise I made to Doc Howell years ago. NEC's growth has not just been about selling enzymes, but rather, it has been about educating the general public and the medical community about the importance of supplemental enzymes to human health.

His mission continues.

And so this book.

CHAPTER 1

A DETECTIVE STORY

It didn't make any sense, Doc Howell thought, as he made his way from bed to bed, from room to room, in the healing environs of the Lindlahr Sanitarium in Elmhurst, Illinois, just outside of Chicago. A week earlier, everyone had been doing fine, drinking their freshly squeezed orange juice and getting their daily butter rubs, and now, suddenly, they weren't. Their gastrointestinal problems were back with a vengeance, as were their skin problems.

Nothing had changed. It didn't make any sense at all. What was going on?

He didn't know it, but at 28, young Edward Howell was about to make medical history.

The year was 1926. It was Howell's first job, and nobody at Henry Lindlahr's "Nature Cure" Sanitarium was taking their job more seriously than this freshly minted MD out of the University of Illinois. Slight of frame and bespectacled, Howell was the son of German immigrants, a scientist to the core, and an iconoclastic thinker. Two childhood surgeries, one to remove his adenoids and another to remove his tonsils, had left him questioning why all children were put through such surgeries at the first sign of inflammation. He could still recall the awful smell of the ether as they placed a mask over his tiny face, then waking up so helpless, the people walking around with surgical masks on. All of this left an indelible mark on Howell and, he would one day tell a friend, made him decide to become a doctor, with the conviction that surgery, while clearly sometimes necessary, should be the very last resort.

And what a time it was to become a doctor.

The 1920s saw some important advances in medicine. Alexander Flemming's discovery of penicillin was huge, though the technology to make this "magic bullet" widely available would not come until World War II. Until then, doctors would have to rely on Paul Ehrlich's very limited antimicrobial drug Salvarsan, which was developed to

treat syphilis. Sulfa drugs didn't come along until the 1930s. And so, in the 1920s, the emphasis was on prevention, on sanitation at hospitals, and at places like the Lindlahr Sanitarium, where entire staffs were devoted to keeping patients as germ-free as possible. Everything got bleached.

The 1920s saw vaccines for diphtheria, pertussis (whooping cough), tetanus and tuberculosis. Frederick Banting and Charles Best's discovery of insulin transformed diabetes from a death sentence into a manageable disease. A number of vitamins were discovered. In 1928, vitamin D became the first commercially synthesized and manufactured vitamin marketed to consumers.

Strides were being made.

On the other hand, tuberculosis was still called "consumption," and there wasn't much doctors could do for the stricken except make them comfortable and see they got lots of rest and a nourishing diet, usually at out-of-the-way sanitariums like the Lindlahr, where plenty of fresh air facilitated prolonged remissions.

The germ theory of disease was barely 40 years old in the 1920s. The immune theory of disease wasn't due until the 1930s, when it would finally help legitimize the allergists, who had been accused of practicing voodoo medicine until then.

Aspirin had been patented in 1900. But it was still the centuries-old opiates that served as the sole reliever of human suffering.

For all its exciting moments, medicine certainly had its limitations during the 1920s, and the 1930s.

On the other side of the coin, naturopathic medicine was going through a growth surge.

ALTERNATIVE THINKING

In its day, which lasted from 1914 until it closed down in 1928, the Lindlahr Sanitarium in Elmhurst became a naturopathic Mecca for more than 80,000 patients worldwide, including three-time presidential Socialist candidate Eugene V. Debs. Its founder, Henry Lindlahr, a wealthy entrepreneur, was inspired to enter medicine after traveling to Germany to take the Kneipp Cure for the diabetes that his American doctors insisted was going to kill him. Father Sebastian Kneipp was a Bavarian priest who reportedly put his own tuberculosis into remission at age 28 by means of hydrotherapy—immersing himself in the icy Danube River several times a week. He was also credited as one of the founders of naturopathic medicine.

As for Henry Lindlahr, following his initial treatment in Europe, which involved hydrotherapy, herbalism, exercise and a diet consisting mostly of fresh fruits and vegetables, he returned to America with his Kneipp regimen, lost 40 pounds and reportedly cured himself of his diabetes. We now know that in many cases weight loss can help Type II diabetics reduce or discontinue their insulin requirements.

After attending the National Medical University of Chicago, he opened his first sanitarium, in Chicago, in 1904, followed by the Lindlahr College of Natural Therapeutics, and finally, the Lindlahr Sanitarium on an eight-acre spread in the country environs of Elmhurst. According to its brochure, the Lindlahr doors were open to people with all manner of chronic and terminal illness—tuberculosis, arthritis, cancer, diabetes—except "those requiring quarantine," and patients who were "violently insane." Patients suffering from a simple "nervous breakdown," however, were not uncommon at the Lindlahr.

In a letter to a prospective patient, Henry Lindlahr wrote:

"We combine in our work everything that is good in the natural methods of treatment, such as pure food diet, hydrotherapy, osteopathy, chiropractic massage, Medical Gymnastics, air and sun baths, Mental Therapeutics,

Homeopathy, and non-poisonous herb remedies. By the judicious combination and application of these natural healing methods, we cure all forms of so-called incurable chronic diseases. Nature Cure knows incurable patients, but no incurable diseases. Any case may proceed to a point where cure becomes impossible, but if there is sufficient vitality to respond to our treatment and the destruction of the vital parts and organs is not too far advanced, a cure is possible."[1]

And "No Surgery. No Drugs."[2]

Basically, Henry Lindlahr believed that chronic disease was the result of the accumulation of waste matter and "poisons" in the body, and that acute disease was Nature's way of cleansing the body. Taking this one step farther, he believed that chronic disease was often the result of the repression of acute disease. So the question becomes: How does one free the body up to cleanse itself of toxins and heal itself? Thus, Henry Lindlahr's "Nature Cure" included periods of fasting with fruit juices, to purge the body of toxins and give it rest and time to heal itself, a vegetarian diet, hydrotherapy, manipulation, lots of exercise and lots of rest. Add to this fever therapy (an age-old tactic whereby body temperature is artificially raised for therapeutic purposes), counseling—Lindlahr

was an ardent believer in the psychoanalytic techniques of Jung and Adler, and the human mind as a source of disease as well as a source of healing—and various detoxifying foods, particularly orange juice, lemon, grapefruit, garlic, bean sprouts, fiber and laxatives.

Then there was butter—fresh from the local dairy—not as a food, but as a topical treatment for all manner of skin conditions, including eczema, psoriasis, allergic reactions, and more. Butter has had a long history of medicinal use. The ancient Greeks and Romans applied butter to their skin to protect it from the sun and keep it lubricated and soft. They also applied butter to their joints to relieve aches, to bruises to promote healing, and to aging skin to make wrinkles disappear. Butter was always present at athletic events. Greek and Roman doctors rubbed it into the areas around broken bones to promote healing. Throughout history, butter has been used as a hydrating lipid salve for many skin ailments, with the belief, although not yet clinically proven, that it might open up clogged lymphatics to help release toxins and promote healing.[3]

And so it was at the Lindlahr Sanitarium. Fresh butter and freshly squeezed orange juice proved to be two of the most healing things young Dr. Howell had ever seen.

Why orange juice for gastrointestinal problems? In the absence of heartburn, indigestion can be caused by a lack of stomach acidity, due to nutritional deficiencies. Fresh squeezed orange juice provides a variety of natural acids, particularly citric and ascorbic acids, as well as key vitamins and nutrients—thiamine, which is important to digestive health, and vitamins C and A, which are powerful antioxidants. Recently, citrus bioflavonoids have been found to enhance and prolong the effects of vitamin C and provide defense against oxidative stress.

The bottom line: several daily glasses of fresh squeezed orange juice, and raw butter applied topically, reportedly worked miracles at the Lindlahr—until the day Doc Howell noticed they had suddenly stopped working. Not only was he seeing no improvement, everybody was getting worse.

THE LIFE ELEMENT

Nothing had been changed, schedule or otherwise. He went through all the charts and couldn't find anything. Why wasn't anybody getting better? That's what he wanted to know, but he couldn't figure it out, not for the life of him.

He was pretty much alone on this one. Henry Lindlahr, who he had so admired as a medical student, had died in 1924, the year Howell had arrived at the sanitarium. In his place was his son, Victor, who Howell saw as the source of growing problems. Victor just wasn't as dedicated as his father, or as passionate. Cost-cutting became the order of the day. Howell watched as the maintenance staff was cut dramatically, at the expense of sanitation. And why buy fresh butter from the local dairy and have the kitchen staff squeezing fresh orange juice three times a day when you can get both products pasteurized from the downtown Chicago suppliers?

That's what the nurse brought to his attention one day. Howell would never have caught it himself. He only saw what came out of the kitchen, patient-ready.

The butter was now pasteurized, as was the orange juice. Both lasted a lot longer than the raw versions. But what did it mean in terms of patient health? How was pasteurization affecting the medical value of these two key Lindlahr staples? Or was it? That's what Howell wanted to know.

Always a voracious reader, Doc Howell read everything medical he could get his hands on, but medical journals were few and far between in the 1920s. So he was constantly corresponding with other physicians and

researchers across the country and around the world—Germany, Switzerland, Japan. That's how you got information in those days. If you heard about a paper, you wrote to the researchers and they would send you a copy. He did it all through correspondence. And that's what he did when the nurse told him that the butter and orange juice were now arriving in Lindlahr's kitchens pasteurized. He went right to the source—in this case, the canning industry scientists—to learn all he could about pasteurization.

And this is where Dr. Edward Howell came to make medical history.

Before pasteurization, every small town had to have its own dairy. Even with refrigeration, milk would go bad in a day or two. Pasteurization changed everything; the shelf life for milk and milk products increased exponentially. Fruit juices too. Shipping became possible and dairies became industrialized. The threat of bovine tuberculosis and other bacterial diseases from drinking milk became much less a matter of public health concern.

But at what price?

What the canning industry scientists told Howell was an eye-opener. Pasteurization, they explained, was a heating process. By heating the milk to 190 degrees for

10 minutes, or to 160 degrees for 20 minutes, they were able to kill what they called the "life element" in the milk, so it would last longer. The same went for orange juice. They weren't just talking about bacteria; they were talking about any life element. That included the natural enzymes in milk and orange juice that cause those two food products to break down and go bad. For the canning industry scientists, the formula for success was simple: the less life element in the milk, orange juice or any canned food, the longer the shelf life. Their mission, they told Howell: to kill off at least 90 percent of the life element.

That's when Howell went into overdrive, trying to figure out how a gain in shelf life could cost butter and orange juice their medical benefit. Basically, what started out as an investigation into the biological basis of the so-called life element in a container of orange juice became a lifelong career.

As it turned out, the canning industry scientists knew a lot about these life elements. They knew they were talking about the enzymes. They knew there were different kinds of enzymes, depending on the food product. They knew that these enzymes deteriorated foods, and also what it took to kill them—i.e., heat. Their intentions were perfectly

good—to give foods a longer shelf life. They had no idea what the effect would be on the consumer, except that the foods would now be safer, without any harmful bacteria. If it hadn't been for Dr. Howell's patients' reactions—or lack of—to these new pasteurized versions of previously raw butter and orange juice, he wouldn't have given it a second thought.

But he did.

Now Howell set out to learn as much as he could about human digestion, and the life element—the enzymes—being lost.

What followed was years of study.

He learned that there were three basic categories of digestive enzymes in our bodies: proteases, which break down protein; amylase, which breaks down carbohydrates (starches and sugars); and lipase, which breaks down fats. Further, he learned that there are enzymes in all living things, and thus everything we eat. Carbohydrate-laden carrots contain amylase; protein and fat-based meats contain protease and lipase, and so on.

STAGES OF DIGESTION

Howell's digestive studies taught him that there were three basic stages to human digestion. The first stage involves the upper, or cardiac, part of the stomach, which he perceived as a holding sack analogous to the first of multiple stomachs, or digestive compartments, in other animals, like the cow, whose stomach is made up of four digestive compartments. The conventional wisdom was that no digestion takes place in the human upper stomach. Not true, Howell learned. Food remains in the cardiac portion of the stomach for approximately one hour. During this time, enzymes in raw foods begin the digestive process. In fact, according to his studies, Howell eventually came to learn that up to 60 percent of digestion takes place in the upper stomach, but only when raw foods are eaten. Cooked foods, just like pasteurized milk and butter, contain no enzymes. Their enzymes are destroyed in the heating process. Hence they contribute nothing to this *predigestive* process.

The second stage of digestion, Howell learned, takes place in the lower stomach, the fundus, where parietal cells in the stomach lining secrete hydrogen and chloride ions to create hydrochloric acid, bringing down the pH

(increasing acidity), and turning pepsinogen into pepsin, which digests proteins. While this is going on, signals are being sent on to the pancreas, letting it know what is coming to the small intestine from the stomach so the pancreas can secrete just the right formula of enzymes, consisting of amylase, protease and lipase—to handle the third and final stage of digestion.

The human body does not make cellulase, which digests fiber. That we have to get from the food we eat, or from supplemental enzymes.

Finally, the digested food passes into the colon, which functions as a fluid dehydration plant, sucking out the liquids and passing the fibrous indigestible material out of the body.

That's the way digestion should work. Unfortunately, Doc Howell learned, it doesn't always work that way. Any accumulation of undigested foods in the colon, due to a lack of enzyme activity along the way, as well as other factors, may putrefy and ferment, killing off friendly bacteria that keep the colon healthy. The adult colon is capable of carrying a large amount of undigested fecal matter—a potentially toxic burden.

Further, incomplete digestion can result in similar toxicity and an immune response in the small intestine,

causing inflammation that can result in "leaky gut" syndrome, which can set off a body-wide inflammatory cascade believed, by some scientists, to increase a person's risk of developing a host of inflammatory diseases, including arthritis, diabetes, heart disease and cancer.

More about all this later.

For now, it's like an automobile engine that doesn't burn gasoline efficiently. All systems suffer.

Knowing what he now knew, the question in Howell's mind became how to get the enzymes—the life element—back into the foods we eat after pasteurization and cooking has destroyed them. This became Howell's lifelong mission.

"I have to do something about this," he told a friend, "because no one knows about it and we are all suffering because of it."

SOLUTION IN HAND

Once again Howell went searching, this time for a source of enzymes to replace what was being lost in the pasteurizing, cooking and processing of foods. If one could get the natural predigestion process going again in

the upper stomach—maybe by providing the right supplement—the human engine would burn a lot cleaner. But where do you begin looking for enzymes for human consumption when hardly anyone even knows what an enzyme is?

Then one of Howell's European connections came up with the name Takamine.

A Japanese-born chemist, Jokichi Takamine became a pioneer in industrial enzymology in the late 1800s when he brought a centuries-old Japanese starch-degrading enzyme technology used in the manufacture of sake, or rice wine, to the American beer and whiskey industry. The Japanese enzyme, derived from fungus, was far more active and easier to prepare than the malt enzyme the American brewers had been using.

In 1894, Takamine was awarded the first microbial enzyme patent in the United States, which he licensed to Parke Davis and Company under the brand name Takadiastase, for the treatment of dyspepsia, or upset stomach, which was thought to be caused by incomplete digestion of starches. The product was hugely successful. Takamine subsequently became a consultant to the pharmaceutical industry.

Then, in 1898, Jokichi Takamine made medical

history in his small laboratory in New York City when he discovered and patented Adrenalin. This revolutionized medicine, in operating rooms by controlling bleeding, as well as in cardiology, obstetrics, and in the treatment of asthma and other allergies.

He would wind up being called the Japanese father of American biotechnology, the Japanese Pasteur, and the Japanese Thomas Edison.

And he was rich, founding Sankyo Pharmaceutical Company of Tokyo, the International Takamine Ferment Company of New York, which manufactured enzymes for industry, and the Takamine Laboratory of Clifton, New Jersey, which manufactured the first true chemotherapeutic agent.

It was Jokichi Takamine who hatched the idea and provided all the funding for the Mayor of Tokyo's goodwill gift of 2,000 cherry trees to Washington, D.C.[4]

Unfortunately, Jokichi Takamine died in 1922, two years before Doc Howell graduated from medical school. Fortunately for Howell, Jokichi Takamine, Jr., the elder Takamine's Yale-educated biochemist son, who had also studied at the Pasteur Institute in Paris, was alive and running things when Howell went looking for enzymes.

By this time, Howell had unhappily left the Lindlahr

Sanitarium, which, under Victor Lindlahr's direction, had fallen into bad graces and was forced to shut down in 1928. Victor would go on to have his own radio show and develop Geritol and the fiber-based laxative product Serutan, making over-the-top, undocumented or unsupported medical claims about the latter that would draw the repeated ire of the Federal Trade Commission, the Food and Drug Administration and the American Medical Association.[5]

By that time, Howell had gone into private practice, and in 1932, with the help of Jokichi Jr., he put together his first enzyme solution, combining an amylase and a protease enzyme provided by Takamine's fermenting operations. Now he had an enzyme supplement that would help digest proteins and carbohydrates. He began giving this powdered enzyme supplement in a little red can to his patients, instructing them to sprinkle it on their food.

And sprinkle they did, with surprising results.

Chronic digestive problems, including diarrhea, reportedly cleared right up, as did skin problems like eczema and psoriasis, as well as food allergies and other health issues. Before long, people started coming to Howell's clinic, not to see him, but just to pick up a can of his powder. A buzz hummed across Chicago. Doctors

started calling him, saying "What's this red can of powder that you've got there? What's in it?" The word spread to other cities and states. In November of 1932, Doc Howell brought in a couple of people and started a mail order operation he called the National Enzyme Company.

And so Doc Howell made medical history. His discovery showed that pasteurizing and cooking foods could deprive us of much of our natural digestive ability, with potentially wide-ranging health consequences, and that enzyme supplementation could restore that ability.

It would take Howell 20 more years to come up with his complete enzyme supplement formula, combining amylase, lipase, protease and cellulase, to aid in all phases of digestion. It was during that year, in 1955, that Howell removed himself from the company. He wanted to remain the pure research scientist, and that's the way he stayed, authoring two books and treating patients. The company would grow in modest increments, remaining a small mail order operation until a young Anthony Collier bought it in 1979 and took it global.

Howell remained the pure scientist right to the end, spending entire days in the library doing his research. At the age of 88, while living in Southwest Florida, he served as Research Director for the Food Enzyme Research

Foundation. Collier, who spent many hours with Howell over the years, recalls him saying one day: "Tony, if it doesn't happen 1,000 out of 1,000 times, it's not proven; and if it hasn't been around for 1,000 years, it's not science."

A TEST OF TIME

Maybe the science of enzymes does go back 1,000 years, or much longer. As we've seen, the ancient Greeks and Romans were aware of the healing powers of enzymes even though they didn't know what they were, or that they even existed. All they knew, *or believed*, was that something in the butter worked miracles on a bunch of medical problems.

Shall we call this intuitive science?

The same was true of other societies that sensed the healing power of fresh vegetables, butter and orange juice, right up to the largely raw vegetarian diet espoused by Father Sebastian Kneipp, and the fresh squeezed doses of orange juice and the daily butter rubs at the Lindlahr Sanitarium.

The science of enzymes has been around for a long time. Looking back, one could say we're just now catching up to history.

That is the mission of this book—to create a greater awareness of the potential power of enzymes and the benefits of enzyme supplementation, as a means of achieving perhaps a healthier and more complete digestion of the foods we eat, and possibly reducing our risk for the array of degenerative diseases shown to be caused by chronic inflammation, including arthritis, diabetes, heart disease and cancer. Studies have now shown that an ongoing factor in this inflammatory cascade in humans is a diet dominated by cooked and processed foods that have little or no enzyme content left in them by the time they are eaten, and are "nutritionally weak."

Even the fresh raw fruits and vegetables that we buy in the supermarket today are losing their enzyme value as the food industry uses new technologies and genetic modification to increase their shelf life.

Again, at what cost?

Doc Howell would know.

There's an even bigger picture here. What we may be looking at is not just the loss of the enzyme content in a stick of butter or a glass of orange juice, but rather the upsetting of the enzyme balance in Nature itself.

It is not the intention of this book to alarm, but rather to educate, and to inform, because each one of us holds the power to change this process in our own lives and in the lives of our loved ones.

One could say the mission of this book is to help restore the natural enzyme balance in human kind, one belly at a time.

Bringing enzyme-rich foods back into your diet, and adding digestive enzyme supplements to your daily regimen, may open the door to a healthier, perhaps even longer life.

On that note, let's move on to enzymes, Nature's Workers.

CHAPTER 2

NATURE'S WORKERS

Okay, so what's an enzyme?

According to the National Human Genome Research Institute, an enzyme is a "biological catalyst," a protein molecule that "speeds up the rate of a specific chemical reaction in the cell." The enzyme is not destroyed during this biochemical reaction; rather, it is used over and over. A cell contains thousands of different enzyme molecules, "each specific to a particular chemical reaction."[1]

That's one way of looking at it.

In Doc Howell's mind, however, enzymes were far more than mere catalysts. Howell saw enzymes as possessing their own "life energy." Like the electricity that

brings life to a light bulb, the enzyme luciferase fires up the lonely firefly in search of a mate.

And so, on a more poetic note, Howell wrote: "I would not like to think, when a person talks to me face to face, that it is the energy of the potato he has just digested that is producing his whimsical remarks and animated conversation. I prefer to believe that complex emotions, such as joy, sorrow, and anger, are powered by the same vital energy that the enzyme complex utilizes in metabolizing food—not by the caloric energy of a potato."[2]

So what are enzymes?

Practically speaking, enzymes are indeed protein molecules that initiate and speed up biochemical reactions in our bodies. More to the point, however, as Howell put it, they are Nature's workers. They are the life force behind the orchestration and regulation of virtually every life function, from the first breath of air we take when we are born and how we utilize that air, to the beating of our hearts, to how we digest our food, to every interaction of neurons in our brains.

Enzymes are the force behind every aspect of life on earth, from the locomotion of a single-celled amoeba, to the coordination of a team of polo players, to the writing of this book.

That's the world as Howell came to see it, with all of life driven by the *Power of Enzymes.*

BASIC ENZYMES

There are three basic types of enzymes.

First, there are the metabolic enzymes, which are involved in every metabolic activity in our bodies. They are, as Howell wrote, "the manual workers that build our body from proteins, carbohydrates and fats, just as construction workers build our homes. You may have all the raw materials with which to build, but without the workers—enzymes—you cannot even begin."[3]

Every organ system, every tissue, every cell has its own workforce of metabolic enzymes to keep it in good repair, running properly, and functioning in perfect harmony with other systems, right down to the synthesis of DNA. And so, phosphorous is fashioned into new bone, the heart maintains its rhythm, blood is oxygenated, our immune systems fight off invaders, waste is removed, damaged tissues are repaired, and so on. The lack of even one

enzyme in the body can mean the difference between life and death.

Howell again: "Metabolism is an enzymic process from beginning to end. Metabolism is Mr. and Mrs. Grandparent Enzyme and their children, grandchildren, great grandchildren and all of their offspring and in-laws, multiplied many times, and all of them ceaselessly at work."[24]

And so we breathe, and so our hearts beat, and so we imagine.

Then there are the digestive enzymes, which convert foods we eat into smaller chemical elements capable of passing through intestinal walls and into the bloodstream, for the nourishing, maintaining and building of new cellular structures.

Digestive enzymes, as discussed in the last chapter, fall into three basic categories: proteases, which break down proteins; lipases, which break down fats; and amylases, which break down starches. They are secreted by the salivary glands, the stomach, the small intestine, and by the pancreas.

Finally, there are the food enzymes that come in the foods we eat. These are enzymes that have lived more than one life. They have provided the energy for the life functions of the organism they were born into, and now they are assisting in its digestion by the organism that has

consumed it. Hence, one organism's metabolic enzymes can become another organism's digestive enzymes—if the life force of those enzymes has not been cooked, pasteurized, processed or genetically modified out of that organism before it was consumed.

Let's adjust the microscope for a closer look.

Enzymes are in fact large protein molecules that contain many smaller molecules, called amino acids, all bound together in amino acid chains. It is the unique configuration of these internal amino acid chains that endows each enzyme molecule with the "charge" it needs to do its specific job. That job might involve breaking down starches into sugars to power the human body. Or it could involve taking carbon dioxide from the air into a leaf, where another enzyme turns the carbon dioxide and water into food to fuel the plant. This is called photosynthesis. The byproduct of photosynthesis, oxygen, is then released into the air for us humans to breathe.

And so all of life is connected through the interaction of enzymes.

There are thousands of different enzymes in the human body, accelerating the biochemical processes that drive every cellular aspect of our lives. Yes, they do this without being altered or used up, though enzymes appear to have a limited

lifespan. And, as Howell noted, our individual longevity seems to be inextricably linked to the life force of the enzymes we carry within us, which diminishes as we age. So it's in our best interest to do whatever we can to preserve our enzyme energy.

For when the light bulb goes out, the light bulb goes out.

MORE ABOUT ENZYMES

Now some fascinating facts about enzymes.

First is their specificity. Each enzyme is designed to interact with a specific substrate, or substance, such as the milk protein casein. Enzymes accomplish this interaction by means of an extremely precise lock and key fit; the enzyme molecule literally docks with its counterpart substrate molecule, at which point the enzyme releases its energy, and the new "product" is created. Further enzyme interactions with other substrates bring about the final objective, whether it's the infusion of a red blood cell with oxygen, the rebuilding of a damaged ligament, or the recognition of a familiar face.

It's all part of an ongoing process—what Drs. Lopez, Williams and Miehlke aptly compare in their book,

Enzymes: The Fountain of Life, to an "assembly line for the step-by-step manufacture of parts and components which are then put together to finally build an automobile."[5]

But on a molecular level!

The speed at which an enzyme works—how fast it converts substrate to the new "product"—is measured in "activity units" and depends on several things.

The first is temperature. Enzyme activity increases as the temperature of its working environment increases. In the human body, enzymes work best at normal body temperature. They become unstable at higher temperatures. When body temperature gets too high, enzymes get fried—they coagulate—and the entire enzyme activity system crashes. It's at this point that the person dies. This is why limbs being transported for transplantation are kept cool—to keep enzyme activity at a minimum, just as one keeps certain foods fresh in a refrigerator.[6]

Another thing affecting enzyme activity is the concentration of the substrate being converted. The greater the concentration of the substrate, the more active the enzymes will become.

Then there's the pH factor. Some enzymes work in an acidic environment while others prefer an alkaline environment. Our pancreatic enzymes do their digestive

work in the alkaline environment of the small intestine, where they are secreted.

Under optimal conditions, enzymes are capable of carrying out up to several million reactions per second.

Finally, enzymes don't work alone. They have helpers, without whom they would be unable to accomplish their individual missions. In his book, *Enzymes: The Key to Health,* Dr. Howard Loomis refers to vitamins and minerals that act as enzyme helpers as the "coenzyme factor." Some act like a "prosthetic" group, completing the enzyme structure so its lock and key fit will be perfect when it docks with its respective substrate. These coenzymes include vitamins B1, B2, B6, B12, and vitamins C and K.[7]

Additionally, many enzymes require metal ion helpers (electrically charged atoms), like magnesium, manganese, zinc, iron and potassium, to activate them—to fire them up. Some helper ions do just the opposite, acting as inhibitors, delaying or terminating enzyme activity.

It's all part of Nature's design. Without inhibitors, runaway enzyme activity could occur in our bodies, resulting in the uncontrolled breakdown of protein. We could literally wind up digesting ourselves!

In the plant world, enzyme inhibitors keep seeds from germinating until conditions are right for them to thrive,

until the acorn has fallen and the ground is warm and moist. It's all part the orchestration of life.

The bottom line: When enzymes are on track, their orchestration defies imagination. The synchronization of enzyme activity within the human body has been likened by Lopez, Williams and Miehlke (hereafter referred to collectively as "Lopez") to "a majestic orchestra conducting a splendid symphony in perfect harmony."[8]

Indeed, let's imagine the human body as a symphony orchestra.

What role would the enzymes be playing? They would be in the stroke of every bow, in the hum of the bass, in the sharp pluck of the harp, in the soaring of the solo violin and in its settling, in the wetting of the reed and in every breath of the woodwinds, in the explosions of brass and in the silences that follow, in every nuance of the conductor's baton, in his body and his eyes, in the beating of every heart, the taking of every breath, in the movement of blood, in the perfect orchestration of the collective.

Just as the human spirit needs music, so does the human body need enzymes.

Given the key role that enzymes play in every aspect of our biological lives, why have they been so overlooked by American medicine? In Europe and other parts of the

world, more than 20 million patients have been treated with various enzymes. American medical students rarely receive any training in enzymology, except for those diseases specifically related to enzyme deficiencies, such as hemophilia. Further, little attention is given to enzyme nutrition or supplements in the possible prevention of disease.

Why has the life force behind all body functions been so ignored?

The answer to this question is best seen by taking a brief look back.

A HIDDEN WORLD

It was the German physiologist Wilhelm Kuhne who originally coined the word "enzyme," in 1876, to characterize a process that had been observed but never understood. Indeed, enzyme-producing bacteria, yeast and fungi had been used for many centuries in the *fermentation* of sugar into alcohol, in the leavening of bread, in the making cheese and yogurt, and in the making of sake and tofu. It's just that nobody knew that enzymes existed inside these bacteria and fungi, let alone that they were the driving force behind this mysterious

biochemical process. Louis Pasteur came close when he concluded that the fermentation of alcohol by yeast was caused by a vital force within the yeast cells, which he called "ferments."[9]

It was the German scientist Eduard Buchner who pinned the tail on the biochemical donkey, when he showed in 1897 that it didn't take an entire yeast cell to ferment alcohol. All it took was an extract from a ruptured yeast cell, which contained the elusive life element itself—in this case, the enzyme zymase.

Suddenly Kuhne's word *enzyme,* which literally means "in yeast," made all the sense in the world.

Buchner received the Nobel Prize and science got its first good look into the hidden world of enzymes. And individual enzymes were henceforth named according to the reaction they carried out, with the suffix "ase" added to the end. For example, the enzyme lactase acts on lactose, or milk sugar, just as lipase acts on fat, which comes from the Greek word lipos, and protease, which acts on protein.

And so, enzymes started taking their place in man's collective mind and vocabulary.

It was right around this time, in 1894, that Jokichi Takamine patented his digestive supplement Takadistase,

which he grew from the fungus Aspergillus oryzae. Takamine, however, wasn't so interested in developing enzymes for medical purposes; he was more interested in the industrial demand for enzymes, which was growing like crazy in the early 20th Century.

So how does one go about mass producing Nature's workers?

The first thing you need to do is find the right microorganism—be it plant or animal, bacterial or fungal, etc.—to produce the specific enzyme for the job you have in mind, whether it's assisting in the human digestion of starches, brewing beer that won't cloud up, as a stain-removing additive for laundry detergents, processing wheat into bread, making cheeses, producing corn and wheat syrups, preparing cotton for weaving, in the manufacture of paper, the tanning of leather, converting corn and other plant materials into biofuels, etc.

It has to be the right enzyme, but not just the right enzyme—it has to be the right enzyme at the right activity level. Because that's how enzymes are measured, not in milligrams like vitamins, but by "activity units." Their potency, their catalytic "kick," if you will.

The search for a specific enzyme often begins with soil sampling that can literally take one around the world.

A single gram of soil contains 4,000 different microorganisms, each capable of producing hundreds, even thousands of different enzymes. It takes about 10 million soil samples to find one enzyme that can be grown commercially.[10]

A daunting task indeed, followed by the equally daunting screening process, which involves purification and growing the candidate fungi in various mediums, or substrates, and under various conditions, and finally testing the enzymes under the exact working conditions in which they are being bred to perform.

All of this is done to identify the mother cell, which is then stored at minus 60 degrees Fahrenheit.

When a batch of enzymes is needed, the mother cell is taken out, warmed up, and put in the right environment, at which point she multiplies, like a queen bee, producing a brood of worker cells. These worker cells are then injected into trays containing wheat, soybran, or the best growth medium to get maximum production out of them. They are then placed in a dark, moist room, much like a room used for growing mushrooms. Within two to four days, a green fungus forms across the top. All that's left to do at this point is separate away the large enzyme

molecules by way of the centrifuge, which literally spins them out of solution.

The enzymes are then purified and combined with a vegetable fiber to render them dry and stable for formulation into the final product.

While the industrial demand for enzymes has created a multi-billion dollar industry, the medical use of enzymes, in the form of enzyme supplements, despite multiple Nobel Prizes and mounting evidence of their benefit to many aspects of our health, as we will see in a later chapter, has not taken off as dramatically as one would expect—not like vitamins did back in the 1920s.

Why did vitamins get attention? Partly because vitamin deficiencies could be linked to specific diseases, and vitamin supplements offered the opportunity for a cure. Such was the case with scurvy and vitamin C, beriberi and vitamin B1, and pellagra and the B vitamin niacin. Science loves instant gratification. So outside of treating specific deficiencies, such as pancreatic insufficiency, mainstream medicine wasn't as interested in investigating and promoting enzyme supplementation.

And unlike drugs, which were measured in milligrams, enzymes were measured in "activity units," which was an alien concept to mainstream physicians.

Also, as medicine grew in America, so did the fear of malpractice suits, along with the tendency to avoid "alternative medicine," particularly in the research community. Further, one cannot patent Nature's drugstore, which makes a billion dollar investment in clinical trials financially impractical. A pharmaceutical company is better off creating a new molecule they can patent.

But something else has been working against enzyme supplementation, and that's medical dogma.

Webster defines dogma as: "A principle or set of principles laid down by an authority as incontrovertibly true."

The perfect example of medical dogma in modern times is the decades of misguided thinking over peptic ulcer disease, which hooks right up with mistaken ideas about enzymes.

Prior to 1982, ulcers arising in the stomach and small intestine were attributed to executive stress, along with spicy foods and excess stomach acid. The treatment? Avoid spicy foods and take antacids, and acid-blocking drugs. This brought sufferers temporary relief from the burning pain of the acid-irritating stomach lining. But as soon as they stopped taking the drugs, people found that the acid would come back and the pain would return with a vengeance.

This went on for decades, until 1981, when a young Australian physician named Barry Marshall teamed up with a pathologist, Robin Warren, who had discovered the H-pylori bacteria in the biopsies of patients who were thought to have cancer. Marshall and Warren tried giving an antibiotic to one such 80-year-old Russian patient in severe pain with this bacteria, and lo and behold, the old man came back symptom-free.

Marshall subsequently started finding the H-pylori bacteria in ulcer patients, one after another.

When he took his findings to medical meetings, he was met with skepticism, even ridicule. Meanwhile, pharmaceutical companies were making billions of dollars on acid-blocking drugs, so they wanted nothing of the idea that stomach ulcers could be cured with antibiotics.

Finally, Marshall did the ultimate experiment. He swallowed a vial of the culprit bacteria. Within five days he was sick to his stomach and getting sicker. After 10 days, an endoscopy revealed H-pylori in full bloom. And when he took a round of antibiotics, he recovered.

By 1985, Barry Marshall was curing virtually anyone with ulcer disease with a course of antibiotics. Other doctors' patients started coming to him, just like they

came to Howell when he started making people well with enzyme supplements.

Finally, the National Institutes of Health put the word out that the young doctor from Australia was onto something. The world finally got the message.

And Marshall and Warren got the Nobel Prize.

Interestingly, the reasoning doctors used to dismiss Marshall—that a bacteria could never survive the acidity of the stomach to take up residence there, or so they reasoned—is the very same reasoning that's been used against Howell's theory of food enzymes. Detractors say that neither food enzymes nor food enzyme supplements could survive the acidity of the stomach long enough to perform any digestive work there. Once again, they have been proven wrong, as we will see in the next chapter.

But medical dogma dies hard.

Looking back, what was needed from the beginning was a person of vision who could take in the big picture, like Marshall, and be prepared to buck the mainstream for decades.

And then along came Howell and his theory of the food enzyme stomach.

CHAPTER 3

THE GATHERING MIND

Dr. Edward Howell's first glimpse of what was to become his life's work in medicine came early in his career.

It occurred just after he arrived at the Lindlahr Sanitarium, before the orange juice and butter debacle, when he observed patients undergoing extended periods of therapeutic fasting experience relief from a variety of chronic ailments—from gastrointestinal and allergy problems to migraine headaches, psoriasis, eczema and other skin issues.

How could starvation make these chronic ailments disappear? It didn't make any sense.

Or did it?

The going theory—and it's a strategy that is sometimes

employed today by doctors treating people in the wake of toxic exposures—was that fasting resulted in a purging of the body's accumulated toxins. To some degree, this was true. But something more had to be at work, and it was.

So begins another detective story.

This is not a book about Doc Howell, per se. Other important minds would come into play as this new field of medicine evolved, and we will visit their work as well. But one cannot write about enzyme nutrition without writing about Howell and his theories and publications, most notably his two books, which pretty much defined the field.[1]

When it comes to the science of enzyme nutrition, Howell was the original gathering mind. He brought it all together. He was the father of food enzymes, and his mind never stopped gathering. Even in retirement, until his death in 1988 at the age of 89, his van could be seen parked outside the Miami library while he sat inside, a pile of 3x5 cards before him, painstakingly recording every new bit of information coming down the pike.

And so it began at the Lindlahr, with Howell's aforementioned odd observation that patients were being relieved of longstanding chronic symptoms while on extended fasts.

How could starvation restore one's health?

The key to answering this question, after years of studying human and wild animal anatomy and physiology, lay in Howell's discovery of the Food Enzyme Concept.

In his words, "The Food Enzyme Concept introduces a new way of looking at disease."[2]

In fact, it was the emergence of an entirely new theory of disease. For what Howell came to see as he looked around him was a world that was "half sick."

And it only appeared to be humans, with their cooked food diet.

"In a biological sense," Howell wrote, "there are no completely healthy people living on the conventional diet. Even those young adults who feel fit have health defects. Some have dental caries, thin hair, approaching baldness, acne or allergies, headaches, impaired vision, constipation, and so on, ad infinitum. And these are just superficial phenomena that the individuals can spot themselves ... What poses as good health today has been aptly termed by one doctor as 'pregnant ill-health,' or the absence of symptoms. Good health as we know it is in reality a prolonged incubation period for a variety of killer and intractable diseases." Those include arthritis, coronary artery disease, autoimmune diseases and cancer.[3]

And yet, he noted at the time, wild animals appeared to be relatively free from these common chronic ailments.

The same was true of zoo animals, if they were eating raw.

That was the bottom line, as Howell came to see it: a belief system that was based on the fact that human beings ate cooked, while the rest of the animal kingdom ate raw.

The missing element, he concluded: food enzymes.

He'd seen it at the Lindlahr, when the healing power was pasteurized out of the orange juice and the butter. And he saw it later, in private practice, as his own patients were relieved of their maladies when he gave them enzyme supplements to replace the food enzymes missing from their diet.

The more his gathering mind took in, the clearer the picture became.

Let's take this chapter and follow Howell's learning curve.

* * *

One cannot talk about food enzymes without talking about the *food enzyme stomach.*

In simple terms, the food enzyme stomach is believed by some scientists to be that place in the digestive system,

be it man or beast (the upper portion of the stomach in humans), where enzymes in the foods eaten—amylase in a carbohydrate-heavy carrot, protease in meat, lipase in avocado, etc.—are used to partially "predigest" those foods. This predigestion by food enzymes lightens the workload down the line for the body's own hardworking enzyme-producing organs, while minimizing the need for disease-fighting white blood cells to be recruited to assist in the more menial task of digestion.

Consider the lion devouring his prey, filling his stomach with as much as 30 pounds of raw meat chunks he has barely chewed, before crawling off to a secluded spot to digest his meal. At this point, cathepsin—the food enzyme in the meat of the prey—goes to work predigesting the meat chunks from the inside. During this predigestive process, as described by Howell, the pressure from the bolus of meat inside the lion's bulging stomach crowds out its own enzymes and acid, while the food enzymes do their work, liquifying the meal.

"Later," he wrote, "pepsin from the lion's stomach juice digests the [remaining] meat chunks from the outside, while the food enzymes continue to digest them from within. Several days may pass before the job is completed."[4]

When it comes to the bird, the food enzyme stomach is

the crop—the expandable muscular pouch near the gullet or throat. While the crop itself has no digestive enzymes, food enzymes are abundant in the seeds and grains the bird consumes. Once in the crop, over a period of 10 to 15 hours, Howell noted, these seeds or grains become moisturized and actually start to germinate. When this happens, inhibitors are neutralized and the enzymes multiply and begin converting starches in the meal into simple sugars. These same food enzymes then pass from the crop to the bird's stomach to further assist in digestion of the meal.

Such is the case with all Nature's creatures, whether their food enzymes come in fruits and vegetables, or in prey. Food enzymes are food enzymes, regardless where they come from.

"There is nothing to prevent the digestive enzymes of the prey from doing the same job in the stomach of their new owner as they did during life for the benefit of their former owner," Howell wrote.[5]

As long as the foods are consumed raw, that is.

Moreover, enzymes, which do not function as digestive enzymes in their "former owner," Howell noted, can become digestive workers when that animal dies or when they are consumed by another animal.

Cathepsin is a perfect example. This enzyme, contained in the muscles and organs of animals, has no digestive function while the animal is alive. After death, however, when the animal's tissues become acidic, protein-digesting cathepsin becomes activated and starts breaking down the dead tissue. And so we all return to the earth.

Cathepsin is also what ages the butcher's beef when it is left hanging in a controlled environment for a prolonged time. So aging is a digestion process—the cathepsin breaks down the protein bonds and you wind up with soft, prime, aged beef.

Or if an animal in the wild happens to consume another, the cathepsin of the prey becomes a working digestive enzyme in the new owner's food enzyme stomach.

And so the enzyme balance in Nature comes full circle.

Cattle and sheep have one stomach with four compartments. Only one of these compartments—the smallest and last in line—actually secretes digestive enzymes. The other three, Howell noted, act as food enzyme stomachs. Like the crop of the bird, they provide a place for the food enzymes to do their predigestive work.

The largest food enzyme stomach in the world is the first of three stomachs belonging to the whale. Dolphins and porpoises, also marine mammals, have this same

digestive setup. The food enzyme stomachs in these creatures secrete no enzymes of their own, or acid. They rely entirely on the enzymes of their prey for digestion—in this case aquatic animals, with seals being a staple of most toothed whales. One killer whale, Howell noted, had 32 seals in its food enzyme stomach when they opened it up.[6]

You would think that such a whale, which dines on large quantities of fat from seals, and is insulated with a thick layer of fat and blubber himself, would be a prime candidate for atherosclerosis—a buildup of cholesterol deposits inside the walls of the arteries. A high-fat diet is a recipe for atherosclerosis in humans.

Not these whales. Their arteries are clean as a whistle.

Dr. Maynard Murray, a marine expert and acquaintance of Howell, dissected between 900 and 1,000 sperm whales, the largest of the toothed whales, in Peru between 1942 and 1945. They were looking for cancers, arteriosclerosis (hardening of the arteries) and arthritis, Murray explained to Howell, but they found none of these common human ailments among these blubber-insulated carnivores that feed on thousands of pounds of fish, octopus and giant squid daily. And when they looked at the whales' arteries under the microscope, they found no cholesterol deposits.[7]

Murray's team also dissected 3,000 seals killed for their fur off the Aleutian Islands of Alaska. Once again there were no malignancies and their arteries were clean.

These were observational studies. They weren't designed to control for variables or anything like that. But many a great discovery in medicine has started out with simple observation.

Moreover, Eskimos whose diet was similar to that of whales and seals also remained relatively free of these common ailments—that is, until they started cooking.

"Before the coming of the airplane," Howell wrote, "the primitive isolated Eskimo was a heavy eater of raw fat and blubber, but paradoxically was acknowledged by medical authorities to be substantially free from heart and blood vessel disease, and most other ailments of civilization."[8]

Doctors going on expeditions to the Arctic, he wrote, "found that the more isolated Eskimos were healthier than those who had extensive contact with traders and missionaries."

One of those physicians, Dr. William Thomas, went on the Macmillan Arctic expedition of 1926 and studied the Northern Greenland Eskimos, who lived remotely and continued to dine prodigiously on raw meat and fish—again a recipe for heart disease. Dr. Thomas examined

142 adults between the ages of 40 and 60 in hospitals with fully equipped laboratories, and he found "no unusual prevalence of vascular or renal disease."

Overall, Thomas concluded, the Northern Greenland Eskimos had "a high measure of good health," leading him to conclude that "an exclusively carnivorous diet does not predispose to renal and vascular disease."[9]

As long as it's raw. For when Thomas compared the "excellent health" of the Northern Greenland Eskimos to the health of the Labrador Eskimos, who dined on the same meat diet, but cooked, as well as dried and canned foods, Howell notes that Thomas found "a distressing situation that has developed with the appearance of a number of diseases." These included rheumatic pain, stiffness of joints, fatigue, scurvy and rickets.

Then there was Dr. Israel Mordecai Rabinowitch of McGill University in Canada, who traveled with the Canadian Eastern Arctic Patrol in 1935, visiting various Eskimo settlements in the Hudson Bay region.

In the northern camps, Eskimos had the least contact with traders and lived on their native raw diet. This included five to 10 pounds of raw meat a day—everything from caribou and buffalo to seal, walrus and whale. Favorite delicacies included the stomach contents of

caribou eaten with seal oil, and clams from the walrus stomach, all of it raw. What a recipe for heart disease! And yet, laboratory analysis of blood samples and blood pressure monitoring revealed no evidence of coronary artery disease or high blood pressure among these raw-eating Eskimos, whereas both were common among the natives in the southern regions who had become civilized and were cooking, as well as using flour.

Nor did he find any diabetes or cancer among the raw-eating Eskimos.[10] When Dr. Rabinowitch published his findings on the health of Eskimos eating raw, in the March 1937 *Journal of Biochemistry*, it made international news, including featured coverage in *Time Magazine*.[11]

The world was fascinated.

For Howell, the conclusion was obvious. "If the raw diet of Eskimos has had nothing to do with their high standards of health and immunity to disease," he wrote in response to naysayers, "how can we explain the poor health and presence of numerous diseases in Eskimos living under identical conditions of climate, but who live near white communities and use a diet more or less extensively cooked?"[12]

The explanation was even more obvious to Howell: It was the fat-degrading lipase and other food enzymes in

the Eskimos' raw diet—just like that of their toothed whale and seal brethren—that kept their arteries clear and their bodies healthier than their more civilized counterparts eating enzyme-deficient foods.

That's what Howell preferred to call them—"enzyme-deficient," as opposed to "cooked," since we know that enzymes are destroyed by heat (i.e., cooking, canning, baking, frying, etc.).

"The secret of the good health of the carnivorous Eskimo," he wrote, "is not that he eats meat, but that he forbids his personal enzymes to digest all of it."[13]

These early Eskimo studies have held up. Dutch researchers recently found a higher risk of heart disease in a cooked "Western" diet than Inuit eating their traditional raw diet.

Dr. Edel Elvevoll, of the University of Tromso in Norway summed it all up in her 2003 review titled, "Impact of Processing on Nutritional Quality of Marine Food Items." She wrote: "Since late 70s, it has been established that Greenland Eskimos living on their traditional marine diet, had a lower incidence of coronary heart disease (CHD) than when living in Denmark on a Western diet."

Taking it one step farther, she adds: "Modern meal-preparing techniques may also lower the content of *biologically* active components."[14]

Biologically active components?

The message is pure Howell: food enzymes are an essential part of life, the food enzyme stomach is meant to be used, and not doing so has its costs in terms of human health.

The story of the Eskimo is the story of humanity, looking back to a time when man lived within the enzyme balance of Nature, taking full advantage of the abundance of raw food enzymes in the world around him, like the rest of Nature's creatures, until he took to fire.

In a 1979 interview, citing fossil evidence, Howell noted that Neanderthal man, who took to cooking his meat some 50,000 years ago, "suffered from fully-developed crippling arthritis."

And so it began.

"Among the thousands of species of creatures living on this earth," Howell wrote, "only humans and some of their domestic animals try to live without food enzymes.[15] And there was no doubt in his mind that enzyme under-nutrition was at the bottom of what he came to regard as man's "health bankruptcy."

Howell never recommended that we consume raw meat or milk. In his day and today, the risk of infection is much too high. His advice to those who enjoy a good steak is to take supplemental digestive enzymes that include strong proteases to help digest the cooked meat.

Knowing also that enzyme production and availability decreases with age—and with the use of certain medications, stress, or a cooked-food diet—it is all the more reason to have enzyme supplements onboard.

It's about putting enzymes (whether from food or supplements) back to work for more complete digestion.

That was Howell's reasoning, and it makes sense.

A PERFECT DESIGN

The physical setup may be different, but the human food enzyme stomach was designed to do the same job as any other food enzyme stomach in the animal kingdom.

Human digestion actually begins before the first bite, with the visual and nasal sensory cues that start us salivating in anticipation of the mouthwatering dish of food being placed before us, or the freshly baked bread emerging from the oven.

Then comes the act of chewing, or mastication. This breaks down the cell walls of the raw foods, releasing the protein, starch, and carbohydrate-digesting food enzymes, while carbohydrate-digesting amylase is secreted by the salivary glands. The process then heads south, down the esophagus and into to the upper or cardiac part of the stomach, which opens up to accommodate the arriving meal.

The cardiac stomach, named for its proximity to the heart, is the human food enzyme stomach, thought by some to be analogous to the first stomach of the whale. There is no peristalsis in this upper cardiac portion of the stomach—no downward-driving muscular constrictions and relaxations. It is here in this holding bin that the meal sits for 30 to 45 minutes, while the acid-secreting lower part of the stomach remains closed to allow the food enzymes from the meal, and amylase from the salivary glands, to do their predigestive work.

Even as the lower part of the stomach opens up and acid levels rise, with hydrochloric acid converting pepsinogen into protein-digesting pepsin, food enzymes are able to continue working. "Even at this point," Howell wrote, "the food enzymes are not inactivated until the acid level becomes prohibitive."[16]

It took a long time for the medical world at large to accept this idea of predigestion. Enzymes are protein-based, many argued, and could never survive the acid environment of the stomach.

Studies have shown otherwise.

At Illinois College of Medicine, Dr. Olaf Bergeim removed foods from the stomachs of 12 dental students 45 minutes after they had eaten. What he found confirmed the digestive ability of the upper stomach: an average 76 percent of the starch of mashed potatoes and 59 percent of the starch from bread had been broken down to maltose, or malt sugar, with an additional percentage converted to dextrose—all predigested.[17]

Surprisingly, 15 minutes was enough time in the stomach for a significant amount of digestion to occur.

This was just from the digestive power of salivary amylase—there were no food enzymes present in the all-carbohydrate cooked meal, and no supplementary enzymes.

Another important study, by Dr. J. M. Beazell at Northwestern University, involved enzyme supplements—amylase, derived from germinating barley. To everyone's surprise, the amylase not only survived the acid in the stomach, where it assisted salivary amylase in the digestion of starches, but 51 percent of this supplemental

enzyme actually made it into the small intestine, to assist pancreatic enzymes in their digestive work.[18]

Further human studies have not been possible in part because modern research regulations typically prohibit stomach pumping in healthy individuals. But there is little doubt left in many scientific minds about the digestive power of the human enzyme stomach.

This is why food enzymes and enzyme supplements, and a healthy diet, are so important. Besides contributing to more complete digestion, which is critical to our health, as we will see, the more food that's predigested, the less work there is presumably for the pancreas to do.

The pancreas is probably the most overworked organ in the human body, as evidenced by its size, relative to body weight, which dwarfs the pancreas size of other animals getting a regular supply of food enzymes in their raw diets.

Moreover, this predigestion is believed, by some scientists, to eliminate the need to recruit the immune system's white blood cells to aid in digestion, at the expense of overall body health and well-being. Having disease fighting white blood cells perform digestive duties, it's been said, is like having Navy Special Forces do janitorial work.

All this came into perfect focus for Howell in 1943,

with a new theory, which he named The Law of Adaptive Secretion of Digestive Enzymes.

And so we continue along the learning curve.

CHALLENGING BABKIN'S THEORY

For the longest time, the scientific world accepted Russian Professor B. P. Babkin's "Theory of Parallel Secretion of Enzymes." Published in 1904, this theory stated, quite simply, that the human pancreas secreted the three main digestive enzymes—amylase, protease and lipase—in the same *strength* regardless of what kinds of food had been eaten. So if you ate a baked potato, besides the amylase needed to digest this carbohydrate food, the pancreas would automatically crank out equal amounts of protease and lipase, even though there was no protein or fat in the meal.

That was the accepted theory, and it made no sense to Howell.

"What kind of physiological law and order would prompt all of the enzymes to be secreted at the same strength when only starchy food is eaten?" he wrote. "One would expect that a baked potato would stimulate only the secretion of amylase, which is the enzyme needed for starch digestion."[19]

And yet, Babkin's theory persisted for decades, despite growing evidence to the contrary.

In Howell's mind, this "false doctrine" set enzyme nutrition back 50 years by encouraging the idea "that enzymes are expendable."

Nothing, in fact, could be further from the truth.

Finally, in 1943, researchers at Northwestern University proved that the pancreas was not that stupid after all. Experimenting on rats, they showed that the pancreas received signals from the stomach, telling it exactly what kinds of foods were on the way, and put together just the right enzyme cocktail to digest that meal.[20]

The findings held up in human studies, most recently in a Polish study published in the *British Journal of Nutrition,* where the pancreas of people in the study reduced production of meat-digesting enzymes when the people switched to an all-vegetarian diet. And then the pancreas ramped up production when the study participants went back to eating meats.[21]

The short of it is that Babkin was replaced with a new improved <u>theory</u> of pancreatic behavior, which Howell had named the "Law of Adaptive Secretion of Digestive Enzymes".

This new understanding also put a big hole in the idea that enzymes are expendable. Far from it, Howell insisted,

"The Law of Adaptive Secretion of Digestive Enzymes holds that the organism values its enzymes highly and will make no more than are needed for the job."

And anything individuals can do to preserve their "enzyme bank account," as Howell called it, such as eating enzyme-rich foods and taking enzyme supplements, will be a boon to their health.

"If you take in outside enzyme reinforcements for predigestion," he wrote, "The Law of Adaptive Secretion of Digestive Enzymes and your food enzyme stomach will become your best friends. They will enable you to allocate fewer of your personal enzymes for digestion and more of them for metabolism. This will keep your whole body operating to make you feel well, prevent disease, and help correct the malfunctions causing human ailments.

"Don't disappoint Nature—give her the outside enzyme reinforcements your primordial ancestors had been getting for millions of years."[22]

That's the way Nature had originally set us up—with the pancreas only putting out enough enzymes to handle the job.

It's all about the body conserving vital energy.

Finally, we arrive at the answer to the question in Howell's mind at the beginning of this chapter—how

extended periods of fasting could make the Lindlahr patients' chronic illnesses reportedly go away.

The answer: Quite simply, Howell deduced, fasting put the entire digestive system on vacation. With nothing to be digested, a patient's pancreas didn't have to supply any digestive enzymes, and, more importantly, disease-fighting white blood cells didn't have to be recruited for digestive duty. Hence, the immune system's Special Forces were free to do what they were meant to do—fight disease and clear away dead and dying tissue from diseased areas.

Moreover, it has been suggested, the digestive vacation that comes with fasting also temporarily reduces the body-wide inflammatory cascade that comes with incomplete digestion and a buildup of toxins.

Anecdotally, this is borne out by people undergoing fasting before colonoscopies—they report feeling much better after the fast. Some scientists even recommend fasting as a household routine to do several times a year to cleanse the digestive system and to optimize health, including a healthy brain. Recent research has reported that occasional fasting not only stimulates the genetic mechanisms for several key nutrients that reduce inflammation, but also can stimulate better brain function.[23]

OUR ENZYME BANK ACCOUNT

This brings us to what Howell called each individual's "enzyme bank account," and the consequences of making too many withdrawals.

Nature's plan, as the theory called the Law of Adaptive Secretion of Digestive Enzymes dictates, calls for food enzymes to assist in digestion, rather than forcing the pancreas and other enzyme secreting organs to become overworked. But when there are no food enzymes to assist, these organs kick in.

"Like an indulgent parent who caters unstintingly to demanding offspring," Howell wrote, "the body responds generously to calls for digestive enzymes. The remarkable thing about the eventual bankruptcy of the enzyme account is that it can proceed quite painlessly, without immediate symptoms."[24]

Without some form of supplementation, Howell cautioned, enzymes are used up with "reckless abandon," leading to enzyme "bankruptcy."[25]

THE CAVEMAN COOKBOOK

For humans, the decline in food enzymes started with cave cooking and evolved over millennia to the modern kitchen, where any significant heat treatment, Howell notes, destroys enzymes. This would include "slow or fast baking, slow or fast boiling, stewing, and frying," all of which "destroy 100 percent of the enzymes in food."[26] Today we know that even if 100 percent of enzymes aren't destroyed in the cooking process, it can be a significant amount, thereby reducing their digestive efficacy.

In his own experiments, Howell determined that immersion in water at 118 degrees Fahrenheit was capable of destroying enzymes within half an hour.

Canned foods require cooking at high heat in order to preserve them. Pasteurization, as we've seen, has done likewise, killing off all "life elements" and increasing shelf life.

This leaves us with fresh fruits and vegetables as our sole source of food enzymes. But here the only rich source of enzymes is in high-calorie produce, like papayas and avocados, while foods low in calories, such as raw salad, vegetables and juicy fruits are low in enzyme content.

With this in mind, Howell constructed a meal: "Let us

say that a certain diet has a value of 2,500 calories each day. If it included a lettuce salad, an apple, and an orange, that would break down into about 200 calories of raw food that supplies enzymes. The calories in the salad dressing must be counted amongst the cooked calories. The result: 2,300 cooked calories that have had all of their enzymes taken from them, and only 200 calories supplying some enzymes."[27]

This assumes that produce making it to our dinner tables is arriving with enzymes intact and fully active. And this is gradually becoming not the case.

Consider the modern harvesting of grain.

Before the combine, harvested stalks of grain were tied together and stood in the fields for weeks, where they would become soaked with rain and dew. Under the heat of the sun, they would begin to germinate and become enzyme rich, before the grain would finally be stripped from the stalks and shipped.

That was then.

"The modern combine harvester," Howell writes, "removes the grain from the stalk immediately after cutting and permits it to be hauled away to the granary. Hence, there is no weathering and consequent enzyme development."[28]

This, Howell notes, is why farmers are having to add enzymes to the feeds of their livestock and poultry.

Then there are the enzyme-targeted strategies the produce industry has developed out of necessity to increase the shelf life of fruits and vegetables, just as pasteurization increased the shelf life of milk.

From the time we stopped buying our fruits and vegetables from local farmers and started buying them in supermarkets, produce distribution has become a race against time, with billions of dollars in overripe produce being thrown out annually. Anything that can help reduce these losses by giving produce a longer shelf life would be welcome to both wholesalers and retailers. Efforts in this area have typically targeted—directly or indirectly—the enzymes that are at the heart of the ripening process.

The ripening process begins in fruits and vegetables with the timely production of ethylene, a gas, which turns on the genes that create the enzymes that cause the fruit to ripen. Basically, the ripening of fruit is a digestion process, with enzymes in the actual fruit doing the digestion. And so you go from a hard, green, somewhat sour banana to a soft, yellow sweet banana.

How does the produce industry control this process?

In the case of the banana, growers pick and ship them green and hard, to avoid bruising. The green bananas can then be placed in a "ripening room" where they are gassed with ethylene, and they begin to ripen. By the time they hit the store, they're ready to eat. We can then put them in our refrigerator to keep the enzymes in check and keep the fruit from becoming overripe before we eat it.

Apples are often placed in a refrigerated warehouse where ethylene is removed from the air to slow the ripening process.

So keeping produce from ripening too quickly involves keeping the fruit cool, keeping the ethylene levels down by means of new packaging techniques, and preventing bruising. Keeping humidity high also slows ripening. One University of California at Davis study found that if you control all four of these factors—temperature, humidity, ethylene exposure and bruising—a peach can last for 28 days, as opposed to just 1 or 2 days.[29]

All this is aimed at reducing enzyme activity, to prevent premature ripening. As a result, there is less enzyme activity in fresh produce by the time it reaches today's consumer than there was in Howell's day.

The latest effort in extending produce shelf life is called TILLING, which stands for Targeting Induced Local Lesions in Genome. This, too, goes after ripening enzymes.

In simple terms, TILLING involves soaking seeds in a chemical, which causes genetic changes, and then breeding the seeds back and forth until the seed with just the right genetic mutation is achieved. At that point, the ripening gene has been "knocked out," and with it, the ripening enzyme.

Arcadia Biosciences of California has been contracted by the Department of Defense to use TILLING to breed long-lasting produce for the military. Besides tomatoes, Arcadia is using TILLING to develop other produce, including lettuce, strawberries and melons.[30]

Without these technologies, much of today's produce would never make it to supermarket shelves with any degree of freshness.

But again, as Doc Howell would say, at what cost?

So we're back to the gradual depletion of the life element in what we eat.

Without supplemental reinforcements, and the right diet, we could all soon be running on empty.

We're close to that now, between pasteurizing, cooking, warehousing and genetic manipulation—and the gradual extinction of your food enzyme stomach, and all that this could imply for one's optimal health.

CHAPTER 4

RUNNING ON EMPTY

It's 11:50 on the morning of May 17, 2001. Dr. Donald Coffey is standing before the nation's top scientists at the National Academy of Sciences meeting on Cancer and the Environment in Washington, D.C.

Numerous other speakers have taken to the lectern for this two-day event, but Coffey is different. From the moment his name was announced, a hush had come over the entire auditorium. Why? Because every time this brilliant maverick with the down-to-earth sense of humor stands up to speak, he surprises everyone. This time will be no different. They all know it.

Coffey is out of Johns Hopkins—one of the nation's most prestigious medical schools. He holds a Ph.D. in

physiological chemistry and is Director of the Brady Urological Research Laboratory at Hopkins. His talk this morning: "Similarities of Prostate and Breast Cancer: Evolution and Diet."

They all sit waiting. And then he does it again.

"What's the only animal in the animal kingdom besides man that gets prostate cancer?" he asks.

He waits, but nobody says a word.

"We have all the zoo records going back, and there's only one animal besides man that gets prostate cancer. Anybody know what it is?"

Nothing. Just a sea of blank faces.

So Coffey tells them.

"It's the domestic dog," he says. "And it goes back to when the dog started eating burnt red meat off the man's table."

Not just meat, but "burnt red meat."

In his quest to understand prostate cancer, Coffey has taken what has been called "a 4 million year detour." Like heart disease, he notes in his writings, prostate cancer "is an illness of fairly recent evolution." While it's been 4 million years since man broke away from the great apes, it's only been 600,000 years since he first started cooking. Man's "wrong turn," in Coffey's mind, took place some 12,000 years ago, when he began eating more processed

meat, when he went from being a hunter-gatherer to a herder-breeder, and to leading a more sedentary life.

"We quit eating a great variety of fresh vegetables and greens from 3,000 types down to about 20," he wrote. "We started smoking our meat, salting it, putting nitrates on it. Now we get everything from the store, nothing from a farm. We call it fresh, but it's not fresh, especially our meat, which most of us prefer well-done, not raw. Everything is cooked."[1]

Sounds like pure Howell.

And right alongside humans down this evolutionary divergence has been the domestic dog.

For his talk at the National Academy of Sciences that day, Coffey focused on both prostate and breast cancer, noting that breasts and prostate glands showed up in mammals at pretty much the same time in history. Coffey sees breast and prostate cancer as "two sides of a coin," in the sense that both occur at up to 10 times the rate in America and European countries than in Asian countries. When the rate of breast cancer is high in a country, so is the rate of prostate cancer, while countries with low rates of prostate cancer also have relatively few cases of breast cancer. And when Asians migrate to Western countries and partake of the Western diet, with its high volume

of cooked meat, their risk of prostate and breast cancer rises accordingly.[2]

Today in America, according to the most recent estimates, one in every six men will be diagnosed with prostate cancer during his lifetime, and one out of every eight women will be diagnosed with breast cancer.

The Western diet. It's the Eskimos all over again.

Poring over zoo records from around the world, Coffey found that "no animal in the zoo as it ages dies from prostate cancer or breast cancer." Zeroing in on prostate cancer, he came across only three cases of cats dying of prostate cancer, while neither horses nor bulls die of prostate cancer, and "only a very few primates have ever died of it. … And the only animal to develop clinical prostate cancer with any significant incidence is the dog—the pet that eats most from our table."

Then came an interesting observation.

Of the two glands that produce the fluid that makes up life-giving semen—the prostate gland and the seminal vesicle—it's the prostate that is prone to cancer, while the seminal vesicle is "remarkably free of prostate cancer." Further, Coffey notes, man is the only meat-eating mammal with seminal vesicles, which are otherwise reserved for vegetarian mammals.

Is this a throwback to man's early vegetarian days? Coffey wonders.

Maybe, he ventures, man was never meant to be a meat-eater after all, let alone an eater of burnt red meat.

Then came the key discovery.

Tucked away in what the Johns Hopkins team has referred to as "a tiny garden of good and evil," deep within the prostate gland, is a "hidden nursery of thousands of stem cell seeds that divide and grow into mature prostate cells." Also within this garden, Coffey's team discovered, is a key enzyme (glutathione-S transferase p), whose job it is to protect these stem cells—to nurture and protect their delicate DNA.

The culprit in the case of prostate cancer, Coffee has found, appears to be inflammation—destructive inflammation—that knocks out the protective enzyme and attacks the DNA of the prostate cells.

"For some reason," Coffey writes, "there's a little auto-immune reaction. And this prostate inflammation makes ... free radicals [highly reactive atoms] ... which attack DNA like crazy."

What does this have to do with diet? In rat studies, Coffey's team was able to control this destructive inflammation by adding enzyme-rich soy in their diets.

So it certainly appears to involve inflammation, and the fact that only man and his dog historically dine on enzyme-deficient cooked meat, and only man and his dog develop prostate cancer.

And certain protective enzymes seem to be the safety valve capable of keeping the inflammatory process under control.

We'll come back to Dr. Coffey's garden of good and evil later in this chapter, with an inflammatory cascade that's breeding a lot more trouble on a much bigger scale.

POTTENGER'S CATS

Prostate cancer aside, one doesn't have to go back 4 million years to see what happens when animals go from eating raw food to a cooked and processed human-style diet.

A look at Pottenger's cats tells the whole story.

His father was the founder of the Pottenger Sanatorium for the treatment of tuberculosis, in Monrovia, California. That's where Francis M. Pottenger started out as a newly minted physician in 1930. His place in history, like Howell's, arrived somewhat surreptitiously. It occurred when he ran low on the cooked meat scraps he had been feeding his

donated laboratory cats and he started feeding them raw meat scraps, including organs, meat and bone, from a local meat-packing plant. Suddenly, cats that had been sickly—many not surviving his experiments, which involved removing their adrenal glands to test the potency of synthetic adrenal hormones he had developed—appeared to be brighter-eyed and in much better health, as did their more vigorous kittens.

And post-surgical mortality went way down.

So begins another detective story, to be played out in Pottenger's 10-year study, from 1932 to 1942, in which he fed three generations of 900 cats either raw or cooked foods, with surprising results.

The cats fed a diet consisting of two-thirds raw meat and one-third raw milk and cod liver oil maintained normal health from one generation to the next, with healthy tissue tone and fur quality. They had good bone health, with optimal levels of calcium and phosphorus, and they were resistant to infection, including fleas and other parasites, and they showed no signs of allergies. They were both friendly and playful, and when dropped from six feet, they landed like cats are supposed to land—gingerly on their feet. Their kittens, born in average litters of five, were healthy with good bodyweight

and nursed in a normal, healthy manner. Miscarriages were rare.

The other group, fed a diet of two-thirds cooked meat, with the same one-third raw milk and cod liver oil, was another story. By the end of the first generation, these cats became lethargic and began developing a host of degenerative diseases. These included heart disease, thyroid problems, vision problems, infections of the kidney, liver, testes, ovaries and the bladder; obesity, arthritis and inflammation of the joints and the nervous system, with paralysis and meningitis.

Unlike the playful raw eaters, they would never purr; they were irritable and nervous, prone to wheezing, sneezing and scratching. X-rays of their bones revealed calcium deficiencies, with bones becoming longer and thinner. By the third generation, their bones had become soft as rubber, then brittle—an inherited condition subject to fractures, and common in humans who eat mostly cooked foods.

By this third generation, cats weren't surviving beyond six months of age. Microscopic examination revealed heavily diseased lungs. Parasitic infections, skin lesions and allergies all increased with each generation, along with persistent diarrhea, pneumonia, miscarriages ... the list goes on.

Actually, just 18 months on the cooked meat diet rendered females unable to give birth to normal kittens.[3]

It would be decades before the culprit in this particular detective story would finally be identified. That culprit turned out to be taurine, which nobody knew was essential for cats. Taurine is a major constituent of bile. While taurine is commonly referred to as an amino acid, technically speaking, it is not. It's derived from cysteine, an essential sulfur-containing amino acid.

Nonetheless, taurine is essential for cats.

Cats need taurine for normal heart muscle function, vision and reproduction. They also use it to form bile salts that aid in digestion. Unlike other mammals, cats are not capable of synthesizing their own taurine from other amino acids. So they must get it in their foods.

Now a key point: Like enzymes, taurine in meats is destroyed during cooking. This is why taurine is added to today's cat foods after the cooking process.

So there was the culprit in Pottenger's studies—or so it seemed.

Like any good detective story, this one has a twist at the end.

And here it is: Even with taurine added to their cooked feline foods, as well as a full complement of essential

vitamins, today's domestic cats still suffer from the same array of chronic illnesses that plague their human and domestic canine counterparts on enzyme-deficient cooked diets. There's obesity, with 25 to 33 percent of all cats either overweight or grossly obese. One in every 200 to 300 cats are diabetic. Kidney failure occurs in three times as many older cats than dogs. Also occurring in cats: hyperthyroidism, hypertension, arthritis, and cancer—lymphoma, leukemia, squamous cell carcinoma, tumors in the lungs, liver, even brain tumors. Then there's pancreatic insufficiency. The treatment? For cats at least: enzyme supplements.

Skin, hair and nail problems are treated with lipase supplements.[4]

And then there were those three cases of prostate cancer Dr. Coffey found in cats.

The bottom line is that enzymes are the essential workers that keep our body's systems working in harmony and in good repair. There is nothing more essential. And when Nature's essential workers are not there to do their jobs, in the foods eaten or through supplements, the result is incomplete digestion, which may produce an inflammatory cascade that can bring an entire zoo to its knees.

AT THE ZOO

In his book, *Food Enzymes: Health and Longevity*, Dr. Howell looked back to a time when animals in captivity were fed a "random diet," especially the carnivores and omnivores. With raw food at a premium, this diet often consisted of large quantities of white bread, boiled potatoes, and cooked meat. "The high mortality rate in past years of valuable zoo animals is well known to those responsible for maintenance of these animals," he wrote. "Reproduction was not often successful and the raising of young a perilous undertaking, especially in carnivora."[5]

Diseases were overwhelming, even at the best of zoos.

From 1901 to 1923, Dr. Herbert Fox conducted nearly 6,000 autopsies on mammals and birds at the Philadelphia Zoological Garden, documenting more than 30 disease conditions common in humans. Among them: acute and chronic gastritis, duodenitis (inflammation of the small intestine), colitis, liver and kidney disease, myocardial degeneration (inflammation of the heart from lack of oxygen), pernicious anemia, arthritis, various cancers, coronary artery disease, thyroid disease, diabetes, gout, pancreatitis and all manner of infectious diseases, often from food contamination. In this wide-ranging study, diet

was determined to be a primary factor contributing ongoing animal illness, death, and failure to reproduce. Other factors included infection and the nature of the confinement—unlike today's zoos, which do their best to recreate the natural habitat, zoos past consisted only of barred cages.[6]

On the matter of diet, even when carnivores were fed raw meat, Fox wrote, they were not fed according to their native diet. Sedentary lions were fed 15 pounds of whatever meat could be obtained at the same time every day, unlike their lifestyle in the wild. And because meat often became contaminated during butchering and storage, a good raw meal was rare. "Many animals are fed vegetable mashes or stews, which can decompose, while bad meat may occasionally be fed," the researchers wrote.[7]

Zoos eventually got smarter in all aspects of wild animal care. And raw became the law of the land. By the time Howell got around to writing his book, two decades later, he was facing a problem of another sort. Suddenly, he couldn't find any animals to autopsy for his organ weight studies, because the deaths among lions and tigers were so few and far between.

Diet was a big part of it.

"Conditions have now changed," he wrote. "Valuable animals are given mostly raw food and little or no heat-treated food," he wrote. "At the Lincoln Park Zoo in Chicago, famous for its low mortality rate, tigers and lions are fed raw meat and bones exclusively with an occasional addition of raw liver. Anthropoids [monkeys/apes] are given bananas, apples, oranges, and raw vegetables. No cooked material of any kind is used.

"The change in the health of captive wild animals has been remarkable. Reproduction and rearing of young are now regularly successful, even among the anthropoids, which are now maintained indefinitely in captivity."[8]

Indeed, today all the carnivores and omnivores at the Smithsonian's National Zoo in Washington, D.C., and at zoos around the country, are fed raw and only raw, containing a full complement of food enzymes.

Researchers studying laboratory animals have come to the same conclusion. One such study was conducted by Dr. Victor G. Heiser, who headed up the Rockefeller Foundation's International Health Board. Heiser got a good look at the health effects of the heat-treated human style diet when he fed it to 2,000 laboratory rats in a 4,000-rat study. The other 2,000 rats got their natural diet. At the end of two years, the rats on the natural diet

were virtually disease-free, while the rats eating the heat-treated diet were afflicted with everything from gout and gastric ulcers to arthritis and tuberculosis.[9]

Studies of this sort have been reproduced over the years with laboratory animals faring equally badly on the heat-treated diet.

As for man's best friend, researchers have been espousing a raw diet for dogs going back to 1934, at the International Canine Congress in Monaco, when 11 papers presented by experts from eight countries declared: "The feeding of dogs should have as its basis raw meat."[10]

Noting similar recommendations from Northwestern University researchers, Howell wrote: "Veterinarians recognize raw meat as indispensable if good physical condition is to be maintained for long periods."[11]

There is a movement towards the raw feeding of dogs today, and those on commercial raw food are reported to be in better health than when they were eating traditional cooked dog food.

This subject, however, remains a bone of contention in the veterinary world, owing to the risk of infection, mostly salmonella and E-coli, so some scientists are against eating raw. <u>With respect to consumption of raw meat by humans, the authors of this book, do not recommend it.</u>

DEAR PANCREAS

So how do we humans fit into all of this? Let's take a look.

The first organ to feel the effects of a heat-treated, enzyme-deficient diet is the pancreas. That's where the responsibility falls for digesting this diet. With no help from food enzymes, the job is not an easy one. Day after day, the human pancreas is called upon to produce more than its intended share of digestive enzymes.

As a result, the human body has one of the largest pancreases, in relation to overall bodyweight, of any mammal in Nature.

Organ enlargement is not restricted to the pancreas. It happens to the heart, when it's forced to work harder to pump blood through arteries narrowed by arteriosclerosis. The increase in size is due to damage of the heart muscle—its walls stretch and thin out—and its ability to pump blood effectively declines. The end result is congestive heart failure. The same can happen to the thyroid gland when it becomes overactive (Graves' disease), producing too much thyroid hormone, or underactive (Hashimoto's disease), or with other conditions that affect the thyroid. Organ enlargement is also common in the prostate and the ovaries. Any way you look at it, organ enlargement is

not a good sign.

The human pancreas is the hardest working pancreas in the animal kingdom.

Howell picked up on this years ago.

"Animals such as cattle and sheep get along with a pancreas about a third as large as ours (figured as a percentage of the body weight) on their raw food diet," he wrote. "Laboratory mice, eating the standard laboratory chow diet of heat-processed, enzyme-free food, have a pancreas two to three times heavier than that of wild mice eating the enzyme diet of raw food they find in Nature. When laboratory rats are put on an enzyme-rich diet of raw food, their pancreas gets only about one-third as heavy as the same gland in rats fed a random diet, or one totally free of enzymes."[12]

In other words, the harder the pancreas works to handle the digestive burden, the bigger it gets.

Here are the actual numbers: an average human weighing 140 pounds has a pancreas weighing between 85 and 90 grams, while the pancreas of sheep weighing 85 pounds weighs only 18 grams. The pancreas of 1,005-pound cattle weighs only 308 grams, and that of horses weighing 1,200 pounds weighs only 330 grams.[13]

When it comes to pancreas size, we humans win hands

down—or lose. An enzyme-deficient diet and an enlarged pancreas go hand in hand. This, and more, has borne out in animal studies. When laboratory rats on an enzyme-deficient diet were permitted to live out their normal lifespan and then dissected, Howell noted, "An astonishing array of typically human degenerative diseases were revealed."[14]

Putting together the human side of this equation, when food enzymes, either in the foods we eat or in supplements, are available to do their work in the upper cardiac stomach—the food enzyme stomach—they are able to predigest up to 60 percent of starches, 30 percent of protein, and 10 percent of fats. That's work the pancreas doesn't have to do.[15]

However, when these enzymes are not present in the foods we eat, and without supplementation, the overworked pancreas may become less efficient, and incomplete digestion may result in an inflammatory cascade that appears to increase our risk of a host of degenerative diseases.

This brings us back to Dr. Coffey's "tiny garden of good and evil."

WAS THE POET RIGHT?

Recapping, what Dr. Coffey's team found when they investigated the prostate cancer link between man and his dog, both of whom dine on "burnt red meat," was "a little immune reaction" in the prostate gland resulting in inflammation. It was that immune reaction, they believed, in the absence of a key protective enzyme (glutathione-S transferase p), that could be the problem. This in turn produced the free radicals that were attacking the genes of the newly developed prostate cells and turning them into cancer cells. Is this the metaphorical "grain of sand" in which the poet William Blake said we might see an entire world?[16]

In some scientists' minds, the answer would be an affirmative *yes*, if we start with the burnt red meat.

In a diet deficient or void of food enzymes, it falls on the pancreas to produce enough digestive enzymes to handle the entire meal, burnt red meat and all. Under these circumstances, with an increasingly overworked pancreas, a failure to achieve complete digestion is sooner or later inevitable. And this is where the potential health problems begin for all of us—in our own little gardens of good and evil.

"Good health depends on good digestion," writes Dr. Howard Loomis in his book, *Enzymes: The Key to Good Health.*

Indeed, when food particles are not adequately digested, they are not able to cross the intestinal wall properly. Continuing down the alimentary canal, they wind up collecting along the intestinal walls—the colon, in particular—"where," Loomis writes, "they putrefy and form toxic chemicals that will be absorbed into the blood."[17]

Many in the scientific community have come to accept this concept. And it's not a good thing, particularly in the case of protein putrefaction—i.e., burnt red meat—which produces a variety of toxins, including ammonia and hydrogen sulfide. These have been associated with ulcerative colitis and colon cancer. The immediate effect of this accumulation of undigested, toxic fecal matter is irritation of the intestinal lining, resulting in gas, heartburn and constipation. The more putrefaction taking place, Loomis notes, "the more constipated the person is."[18] Enzyme-packing white blood cells come in to help digest and clean up the toxic mess.

And so the inflammatory process begins.

Then there's the threat to the friendly bacteria that reside in the colon. This includes thousands of different

bacterial species that play an important role in helping maintain *homeostasis,* or a healthy environment in the bowel, which includes assisting in everything from carbohydrate and protein digestion, to maintaining the integrity of the intestinal lining, to helping the immune system deal with a variety of harmful organisms that find their way into the gut. Some of the byproducts of these bacteria are also useful, such as vitamin K, which is necessary for coagulation of blood.

Basically, in the colon, there are so-called friendly bacteria and unfriendly bacteria, including other organisms like fungi, or yeast. Like any living cells, these organisms must feed, and they do so in the colon, on foods that have not been entirely processed, or digested. After feeding, they discard their own waste back into the environment, or the bowel in this case.

Now here's the rub. The waste discarded by the unfriendly bacteria is alkaline forming. The more alkaline the colonic environment becomes, the more constipated you become. On the other hand, the so-called friendly bacteria discard waste that is acidic. That's a good thing in the colon. This is how friendly bacteria help maintain a healthy pH in the bowel. There's a symbiotic relationship between these "friendlies" in need of nourishment, and

the colon, which in turn benefits from their presence. Any toxic threat to the friendly bacteria is a threat to the healthy digestive environment in the colon.

With the "unfriendlies," it can be just the opposite. When homeostasis is upset, when inflammation occurs, that's when the unfriendly bacteria start multiplying like crazy. When the environment is homeostatic, and everything is cool, the unfriendly bacteria lie low and don't cause any trouble.

Any way you cut it, as Loomis notes, "maintenance of a normal bacterial flora is imperative for health."[19]

Taking this one step further, when things get toxic and the integrity of the intestinal wall becomes compromised, the result is "leaky gut" syndrome, where toxins and partially digested food molecules cross into the lymphatic system and the blood stream and wreak havoc throughout the body, causing a myriad of inflammatory problems before they can be detoxified by the liver. Leaky gut is thought to play a role in children with autism; they sometimes suffer from digestion problems due to possible food intolerances. In recent studies, researchers have been using these enzyme supplements with surprising success as we will see in Chapter 6. Initial results show that the children's digestive problems have improved as well as

some of their behavioral issues, which often stem, as many scientists believe, from food intolerances. In Chapter 6, we will address this in detail.

The important point here is that complete digestion of the foods we eat is essential to the health of our digestive system, and the rest of our body, as we will soon see.

So there's your garden of good and evil, so to speak—deep inside the human body, where the final stages of digestion occur. But unlike the inflammatory problems Coffey found in the prostate, those occurring in the colon are not confined to the colon, which is why undigested, putrefying food may play a larger role in the process of inflammation, and may lead to arthritis, heart disease, and a host of other degenerative and destructive diseases, including cancers, and, yes, prostate cancer.

What we're talking about involves the immune system. It's called digestive leukocytosis, which involves the mobilization of millions of white blood cells, and the formation of circulating immune complexes that result in body-wide inflammation.

So let's take a look at the big picture.

CHAPTER 5

THE BIG PICTURE

On July 27, 1988, the Surgeon General's office came out with its Report on Nutrition and Health. It was a landmark event, in that it documented our arrival as a fast-food nation, with all the negative health consequences associated with a high-fat, high-sugar diet, "often at the expense of foods high in complex carbohydrates and fiber—such as vegetables, fruits and whole grain products."[1]

"What we eat," the report stated, "may affect our risk for several of the leading causes of death for Americans, notably, coronary heart disease, stroke, atherosclerosis, diabetes, and some types of cancer. These disorders together now account for more than two-thirds of all deaths in the United States."

Not to mention the obesity epidemic.

While under-nutrition "remains a problem in several parts of the world, as well as for certain Americans," the report went on, "for most of us the more likely problem has become one of overeating—too many calories for our activity levels and an imbalance in the nutrients consumed along with them."

Certain groups in the population—"poor and minority groups"—were reaching critical mass in terms of obesity, high blood pressure, and adult-onset diabetes mellitus, which "is strongly associated with obesity."

Between 20 and 50 percent of adults in many Native American tribes, the report estimated, had been diagnosed with diabetes. Navajo children were being diagnosed as young as eight years old!

That was 1988. In the past 25 years, it's only gotten worse!

Where was it all coming from?

The obvious sources: convenience stores and fast-food chains were popping up like crazy outside reservations, and everywhere else, churning out high-fat foods, like burgers and fries, and pushing 16- to 44-ounce cups of soda pop, the latter containing the equivalent of 55 sugar cubes.

That and increased alcohol consumption.

And it wasn't just Native Americans and minority

groups. The Surgeon General was ringing the alarm for all Americans.

The recommendations:

Reduce consumption of fat (especially saturated fat) and cholesterol, and increase consumption of complete carbohydrates, including fresh vegetables, fruits, whole grain foods and cereal products. Eat fish, poultry, lean meats, and low-fat dairy products.

"Use preparation methods that add little or no fat."

Cut down on sugar and sodium, go easy on the alcohol, and match caloric intake with energy expenditure to achieve and maintain desirable body weight.

In other words, don't eat more than you can burn.

And ease up on the red meat.

Basically, consume less of the bad stuff, more of the good stuff, and be healthy.

It was good advice for the fast-food nation.

And yet, another side of the story was not being told.

The Surgeon General's Report had focused on what and how much we consume, as it relates to obesity, heart disease, stroke, atherosclerosis, diabetes, cancer and so on.

The other side of this equation is how much we don't digest.

Note that the word enzyme/enzymes appears 97 times in the 750-page Surgeon General's Report. The historical identification of digestive enzymes is even credited as being the beginning of "modern digestive physiology."

And yet, at no point in the report is there a reference to food enzymes, or to foods high in enzymes that might aid in digestion.

It's not only *what* or *how* much we eat that is driving this inflammatory cascade and the epidemic increase in the aforementioned disease conditions. It's about digestion. And this is where enzymes can play a critical role.

So let's take a look at this health crisis from the perspective of incomplete digestion.

OUR IMMUNE SYSTEM VS. INCOMPLETE DIGESTION

In the best of all possible worlds, our immune system would be able to handle any and all problems—viruses, bacteria, you name it. But like any good system, it has its limitations. Such is the case when we fail to properly digest all the food we eat, and our immune system may wind up with more work than it was intended to handle.

Imagine, if you will, the orchestral goings on in the

colon as friendly and unfriendly bacteria feed on the undigested remnants of a thoroughly satisfying meal consisting of steak and potatoes broiled and baked to perfection. The extra work in digesting this enzyme-deficient meal almost seems worth it as the mind drifts back, savoring the immediate past of the aromatic feast.

Almost worth it, that is, because even as bacteria and other organisms feed on the undigested remnants of the meal, and the mind drifts back, a toxic environment may be in the making.

The trouble, Dr. Loomis notes in *Enzymes: The Key to Health*, actually starts in the small intestine. Food particles, digested to the point where they are small enough to make their way through the intestinal wall and into the bloodstream, may not be small enough to be used by the body's cells. Those partially digested food particles crossing into the bloodstream are regarded as foreign antigens, setting off an immune response.

Food particles not small enough to pass through the intestinal wall continue down into the large intestine, Loomis continues, but not before being fed upon by unfriendly bacteria residing in the ileum, the last part of the small intestine. As they feed, these foraging bacteria release their own digestive toxins into the environment.

This process continues into the large intestine, with an exponential increase in the unfriendly population, as the immune system's white blood cells respond and do their best to clean up what is becoming an increasingly toxic mess.

All this toxicity and activity causes irritation and inflammation of the intestinal wall, to the point where the undigested food particles, as well as the bacterial toxins, can now cross the "leaky bowel" and enter the bloodstream and the lymphatic system.

These blood-borne irritants, as Dr. Loomis has pointed out, can "cause a number of inflammatory problems before they can be detoxified by the liver."[2]

HOW BAD CAN IT GET?

The symptoms of "intestinal toxemia" alone, according to Dr. Loomis, include skin, hair and nail problems (eczema, psoriasis, etc.), sinus and inner ear problems, eye strain, irregular beating of the heart, arthritis, fibromyalgia, and a wide range of gastrointestinal and nervous system symptoms, including depression, irritability, loss of concentration, poor coordination, and loss of memory.[3]

That's part of the picture; the other part is a thing called digestive *leukocytosis*, which involves the immune system's white blood cells.

Simply put, the word *leukocytosis* refers to an increase in the number of disease-fighting white blood cells, or leukocytes, in a person's blood. Usually it's the immune system mobilizing its troops in response to a viral or bacterial infection, though leukocytosis can also occur after strenuous exercise, as a result of emotional stress, or during pregnancy and labor, allergic reactions, or incomplete digestion. Any one of these things may cause the number of white cells in our blood to go up.[4]

When it appears to occur in response to incomplete digestion, it's called digestive leukocytosis.

The first to discover that the number of white blood cells in circulation varies was the Dutch ophthalmologist Franciscus Donders, in 1846. Donders was a pioneer in the field of ophthalmology. He was also a student of general physiology, of evolution, and the way blood flows and oxygen is utilized in the brain. His discovery that the number of white blood cells is not constant proved to be way ahead of its time—the field of immunology wasn't born until the 1930s.

The German physician Rudolph Carl Virchow was first

to describe *digestive* leukocytosis, whereby the number of white blood cells goes up after a meal. Virchow didn't see anything to be concerned about, though, because this rise in white blood cell numbers occurred in every one of his study participants after eating.

So it was perfectly normal, right?

Not necessarily.

It was three decades later that Dr. Paul Kouchakoff, of the Institute of Clinical Chemistry in Lausanne, Switzerland, came forth with studies suggesting that there was nothing normal about digestive leukocytosis after all. Dr. Kouchakoff started his presentation at the First International Congress of Microbiology in Paris in 1930 by explaining that "The living organism is very sensitive to all harmful influences and reacts against them immediately." Hence the increase in the number of white blood cells during "simple and infectious illness, when extraneous [foreign] substances are introduced into our system."[5]

No surprises there.

He explained how researchers have noted this rise in white cells occurring after meals.

Then came the bombshell.

He told them that his team had observed no such rise

in white blood cells after raw meals, only cooked.

Between 1928 and 1930, Dr. Kouchakoff's team had taken thousands of blood samples after people had eaten three different types of foods:

1. Natural raw foods, which had undergone no preparation whatsoever before they were consumed. These included foods like fresh vegetables, raw honey, raw eggs, raw meat, raw fish, fresh milk and butter—"In other words," he wrote, "foodstuffs in the state in which they exist in Nature."
2. Cooked foods, which consisted of natural foods that had been "altered by means of high heat."
3. Manufactured foods—things like sugar, wine, vinegar, and chocolate.

With the natural, uncooked foods, there was no leukocytosis—no jump in the number of white blood cells—while the cooked natural foods produced a rise in the white cell count as if a bacteria, virus or other foreign invader had entered the person's body. Pressure cooked foods also produced a jump in white cells, as did the factory-produced foods, especially wine, sugar and vinegar.

Cooked, smoked and salted animal flesh brought the biggest jump.

Leukocytosis, he reported, occurred as early as 3 to 5

minutes after eating began, it typically peaked at about 30 minutes, and the white blood cell counts returned to normal by 90 minutes.

Dr. Kouchakoff published his findings in 1937. The title of the article: "New Laws of Human Digestion Based on Digestive Leukocytosis."[6] Kouchakoff's conclusion: "We can change our blood formula in the direction we desire by dieting."

Or so he theorized.

Add enzymes to the picture and a new theory of digestion—or lack of it—emerges: Digestive leukocytosis is the immune system mobilizing its white blood cells to pick up where the body's own digestive enzymes fall short, breaking down and hauling off undigested food fragments along with toxic bacterial waste.

Add Howell's work on food enzymes and the emerging theory takes on yet another dimension: Without the predigestive work of natural food enzymes, this is what we are left with—partially digested foods, growing toxicity, an immune response to clean up the mess, and an inflammatory cascade that may result in a wide range of degenerative diseases.

AHEAD OF HIS TIME

It appears that many of Howell's observations may actually be correct with respect to incomplete digestion as a possible source of inflammation.

Some scientists now agree that undigested food fragments in the intestines, in the blood, and elsewhere in the body, are perceived as "foreign antigens," and like other antigens, such as bacteria and viruses, they are capable of causing an inflammatory immune reaction.[6,7] This is where digestive enzyme supplements come in. By facilitating more complete digestion, they have the potential to reduce the presence of these partially digestive food particles and the body's inflammatory immune reaction to them. It's also believed that inflammation plays an important role in the cause of most, if not all, chronic degenerative diseases, from arthritis and cardiovascular disease to Alzheimer's disease, chronic kidney disease, type 2 diabetes and cancer. So if we can reduce inflammation by adding enzyme supplements to a diet of healthy food, we may be able to reduce our risk of developing these inflammatory diseases.[8]

In basic terms, acute inflammation begins when the immune system's white blood cells mobilize and

take action against something foreign that needs to be eliminated from the body, like a bacteria or virus—an antigen. The symptoms of acute inflammation include: pain, heat, swelling and redness. All this is believed to be from the heat of battle, with increased blood flow and white blood cells entering the area of conflict.

Chronic inflammation, which involves the same cellular players, may be more subtle, in terms of symptoms, until it results in chronic disease, at which point there's nothing subtle about it.

Let's take a look at these players.

Generally speaking, there are different types of white blood cells. The granular leukocytes contain enzyme packages to break down engulfed viruses, bacteria, waste material, and so on. Then there are nongranular lymphocytes, which produce antibodies capable of neutralizing bacteria and viruses, and monocytes. These monocytes swell up and transform into enzyme-packing macrophages when they arrive at an area of infection.

Macrophages are the immune system's sanitation workers, capable of engulfing, digesting and hauling off much larger and greater numbers of antigens—micro-organisms and foreign particles, as well as damaged body cells or cells that have run their course and are no longer

useful, and cancer cells and dead tissue.

When it comes to gobbling up undigested food particles, size counts and macrophages are king.

Looking at the big picture, we all live in what might be regarded as a sea of intracellular and extracellular fluids. The insides of our body cells are filled with fluids. This is each cell's internal environment, where it makes its energy and carries on various functions. At the same time, all of our body cells are surrounded by a sea of fluids, which brings them nourishment and takes away their metabolic wastes, to be eliminated by the kidneys. Blood, lymphatic fluids, hormonal juices, it's all part of this sea of extracellular fluids where everything is connected, just like we are all connected by the air we breathe, and the rain that falls in our gardens.

And just as the air and the rain can become toxic, so too can the extracellular fluids in our bodies become toxic.

With incomplete or *improper* digestion, inflammation can start in the intestines, as white blood cells respond to clean up what has become a toxic mess, gobbling up undigested food particles, dead tissue, etc. The effort at this point in the battle is to keep these food antigens from crossing the intestinal barrier and entering the body. Unfortunately, as the battle ensues, the intestinal wall can

become irritated, then inflamed and "leaky," opening the way for these partially digested food particles, as well as bacterial toxins, to enter the blood stream and the lymphatic system.

And so the inflammation can spread. Once in the bloodstream, partially digested food "antigens" are greeted by antibodies created by lymphocytes. These antibodies bind to the food particles, forming what are called *circulating immune complexes,* which can be recognized by macrophages on the hunt. Immune complexes not detected and consumed by macrophages *may* continue to circulate until the blood or other fluids become overloaded, at which point and they begin settling on the surfaces of surrounding cells.[9]

These immune complexes fall like toxic rain onto cell surfaces. It could be cells inside the artery walls, cells in the joints, or cells in the prostate gland—Dr. Coffey's "little garden of good and evil."

How else would burnt red meat find its way into the prostate gland?

And it's not just the immune complexes. Bacterial toxins from the leaky digestive tract are also making their way around the body via this extracellular mainstream.

Each cell has its own means of dealing with immune complexes that come to reside on its surface. Inside the

cell are little pockets of enzymes, called lysosomes, which migrate to the inner surface of the cell and regurgitate their enzymes through the membrane to the outside of the cell where they digest the foreign matter.

Sounds good.

And yet, everywhere this protective process occurs—in joints, on the inside of artery walls, in the kidneys, on any and every cell surface inside the body, in every corporeal nook and cranny, in every tiny garden of good and evil—inflammation and tissue destruction are inevitable.

Add to this a second-wave response of protein molecules whose job it is to assist the existing troops in the war effort by "bursting" unwanted cells and further marking antigens for destruction by macrophages. Now the inflammatory picture is complete.[10]

All this activity—cells attacking immune complexes on their surfaces, macrophages gobbling up and hauling off as much digestive waste as possible, the second-defense wave of proteins joining in the attack, and circulating bacterial toxins—can potentially result in chronic inflammation and tissue destruction.

Continuing inflammation like this can be very taxing on the immune system, and the body's enzyme supply.

"The primary response to inflammation is by the immune system and its increased use of enzymes," Loomis writes. "Localized deficiencies of enzymes can prolong inflammation and delay healing. It has been reported the oral use of supplemental proteolyic enzymes can reduce healing times by up to 50%."[11]

We'll take an in-depth look at the therapeutic use of supplemental enzymes in the next chapter.

FROM INFLAMMATION TO CHRONIC ILLNESS

So how do we go from inflammation to chronic disease?

It starts when acute inflammation becomes chronic inflammation.

In most cases, inflammation occurs when our immune system mounts an attack against an antigen. Once the bacteria or virus is eliminated and the area is cleaned up, redness, heat, swelling, and pain subside, and everything hopefully returns to healthy normal. However, when antigens persist, or when they just keep coming, acute inflammation can become chronic inflammation.

With a continuous stream of undigested food particles coming down the intestinal pike, potentially finding their

way across the intestinal barrier into the sea of extracellular fluids, the immune system remains in a state of constant response.

Wherever these food antigens and bacterial toxins persist, the battle continues, and there is inflammation. It can continue for a long time, at a very low level with no symptoms, until the symptoms of a developing disease appear.

One of these silent killers is high blood pressure. Another is rheumatoid arthritis, which is an inflammatory cascade that can affect different tissues and organs. This disease usually occurs in the more flexible *synovial* joints. The small joints of the hands and feet are the most commonly involved. However, larger joints—shoulders, knees, etc.—can also become affected. In the most severe cases, the pain can be body-wide and disabling.

It starts with inflammation—swelling of the cells that make up the synovial membrane that encapsulates our joints and secretes the fluid that lubricates these joints. As the synovial membrane becomes inflamed and thickens, the joints become swollen, tender and warm, and they fill with excessive fluid. As the disease progresses, the surface of the joints, the cartilage, becomes eroded, further restricting movement. In some cases, this can result in deformity.

Treatments include physical therapy, occupational therapy and nutritional therapy, none of which do anything to slow down the progression of joint destruction. Aspirin and other anti-inflammatory drugs and steroids relieve symptoms, but they don't slow down joint destruction either. The only thing in this country that has been shown to slow progression of rheumatoid arthritis are so-called "disease modifying drugs," which act on the immune system. This includes injection of gold preparations. Unfortunately, many of these medications may have limited benefit and carry potentially serious side effects.

So we're back to the immune system, though the exact mechanism driving rheumatoid arthritis remains something of a mystery.

And yet, we're not entirely in the dark.

We do know that rheumatoid arthritis starts with inflammation of the synovial cells, which secrete the synovial fluid that lubricates our joints. These cells are bathed in synovial fluid, which is part of the extracellular sea of fluids.

Studies have shown that people with rheumatoid arthritis have circulating immune complexes in their blood and in the fluid in their rheumatic joints. One recent study found higher levels of circulating immune

complexes in the joints of rheumatoid arthritis patients than people without rheumatoid arthritis. Bacterial endotoxins have also been found in rheumatic joints.[12]

So all the elements are there. Could this be the toxic rain falling on the synovial cells that is causing them to become inflamed and making joints arthritic?

And could it be diet-related—at least partially?

If this is the case, the best way to deal with the inflammation of rheumatoid arthritis might be preventive. If we were to more completely digest what we eat, some scientists believe, there might be fewer circulating immune complexes and bacterial toxins making rounds in our bodies.

It's an interesting thought.

Because wherever the toxic rain falls, inflammation appears to be inevitable.

Circulating immune complexes settling onto cells in the kidneys result in glomerulonephritis, inflammation of the filters that remove excess fluid and waste from the bloodstream.[13]

Studies have shown that these complexes can also cause pulmonary fibrosis and pancreatitis—both inflammatory conditions. They have also been implicated in lupus and atherosclerosis.[14]

Why atherosclerosis?

First off, metabolic enzymes play an important role in keeping our blood vessel walls clean, breaking down cholesterol and various debris from the bloodstream, as well as keeping our blood fluid. That's what the enzyme plasminogen does. When it's converted into its active form, plasmin, it dissolves blood clots.

One of the biggest advances in medicine in recent years involved the development of a life-saving drug called tissue-type plasminogen activator, or TPA. By injecting this clot-busting enzyme drug into the bloodstream, emergency department doctors are able to dissolve away life-threatening blood clots and restore blood flow in people having heart attacks and strokes. This has been a huge life-saver, as well as sparing stroke victims lifelong disabilities.

If only it were that easy to clean plaque off narrowing artery walls.

Our arteries are prone to narrowing, when cholesterol crystals floating in the blood attach to the inside of the artery walls and white blood cells combine with these crystals to form plaque. This is the start of atherosclerosis. Then come the circulating immune complexes and macrophages, and inflammation begets inflammation.

Recent studies have shown that the mere presence of circulating immune complexes in a person's blood is a reliable indicator of atherosclerosis. And a person's risk of having a heart attack by age 70 may actually to some degree be predicted based on the amount of circulating immune complexes in his or her blood at age 50.[15]

Dr. Clett Erridge at the University of Leicester in England has traced the development of atherosclerosis directly to the foods we eat. He calls what he has found PAMPs, or "pathogen-associated molecular patterns," which refers to molecules "which can be potent inducers of inflammatory signaling."[16]

In other words, these PAMP molecules initiate inflammation.

PAMPs circulating in the blood can come from chronic infections and from the friendly bacteria living in our intestines. But the primary source of these circulating PAMPs appear to be enzyme-lacking processed foods, including processed meats and pre-prepared foods, according to some scientists.

All of these foods contain PAMPs, which are absorbed into the body and can promote inflammation.

So there's another piece of the inflammatory puzzle, this one traced directly to the enzyme-deficient processed

foods we eat—foods that Howell and others long ago tagged as disease-causing inflammatory troublemakers.

None of this is of any significance to the whales, of course, whose fatty foods are eaten raw and come with a full complement of fat-digesting lipase.

The whales also appear to be immune to the cancer epidemic, which brings us back to Dr. Coffey's little garden of good and evil.

MORE ABOUT INFLAMMATION

There's little doubt in anybody's mind that inflammation is a big player in the development of cancer. And now burnt red meat has become an official culprit.[17]

A recent study by University of Southern California researchers found that red meats cooked at "high temperatures" (pan fried or well done) are associated with prostate cancer.[18]

Dr. Coffey, however, holds the distinction of pairing man and his domestic dog in this shared risk. Dr. Coffey also gets credit for coming up with a glimpse at the mechanism—the missing protective enzyme and the resulting inflammation and free radical attack on the

DNA of new prostate cells, turning them cancerous.

Cooked red meat, researchers found, especially processed (cured) red meats like hot dogs, bologna, sausages and bacon, have been implicated in colorectal cancer and esophageal cancer.[19]

In another study, the risk for colorectal cancer actually increased by 21 percent for every 50 grams of processed red meat people ate per day, and by 29 percent for every 100 grams they ate per day.[20]

In other studies, processed meats have been associated with bladder cancer.[21] Cooked red meat has also been linked to kidney cancer.[22] Finally, a "high intake" of cooked red meat has been found to raise the risk for lung cancer by 35 percent.[23]

So what's going on?

Simply put, cooked and processed meats are known antigens capable of sparking an immune response and the resulting inflammation. Add to this the free radicals attacking DNA, and you've got normal cells turning into cancer cells wherever the toxic rain falls.

And it's not just about cancer.

In a recent European study, involving a half million people followed for 12.7 years, those who ate a lot of processed meat had a higher overall mortality rate—a 43 percent higher death rate from cancer, and a 70 percent higher death rate from heart disease.[24]

According to the researchers: "Mortality increases with increasing amounts of processed meat consumed."

An American study found the same thing—an increased mortality rate among people eating red meat. Cooked red meat. They also found that replacing red meat with other healthy foods reduced mortality rates.[25]

Seems like the Surgeon General's advice was right.

Of course, we'd all be even better off without the undigested food antigen problem. That's the other side of the equation.

And if we eat more wisely, of course.

One thing appears certain: Without the constant flow of undigested food antigens and bacterial toxins making their way around our bodies, triggering immune responses and inflammation wherever they settle, we'd probably be a whole lot healthier and less at risk for a host of diseases.

We may even have a shot at living longer lives.

That's the big picture.

And that's where digestive enzyme supplements and healthy foods may just play a role, as we will see in the next chapter.

CHAPTER 6

"ENZYMES TO THE RESCUE"

—Dr. Edward Howell

Can enzyme supplements along with the right foods really help us live longer?

That's what Doc Howell believed, and he wasn't alone in this thinking.

Howell believed that we are all born with an ability to generate the enzyme energy we need to drive all our life functions. New enzymes are constantly being created by body cells to replace those that have "worn out" and been eliminated. Like the energy supply in a new battery, the enzyme energy we are born with—our "enzyme potential," Howell called it—and our ability to create sufficient numbers of new enzymes to maintain this potential, must last us a lifetime.

That means from the day we are born until the day we die.

A number of things can affect our enzyme potential. Enzyme production goes down, for instance, when we're under stress, whether it's psychological stress or the physical stress one experiences as a result of, say, surgery. Certain medications can affect enzyme production. Enzyme production also decreases as we age. Then there's the burden an enzyme-deficient diet places on our pancreas and other enzyme-producing organs over a lifetime.

Hence, whatever we can do to preserve our enzyme potential, Howell came to believe, should pay off in terms of longevity. That included eating enzyme-rich foods and taking enzyme supplements.

That was Howell's reasoning. And it was not entirely without scientific basis.

In the 1930s and 1940s, researchers at Michael Reese Hospital in Chicago measured digestive enzymes in people ranging in age from 12 to 96. The enzymes pepsin and trypsin in the older people were one-fourth that of the strength of the same enzymes in the younger people. Salivary amylase was 30 times stronger in young adults than in people over age 69.[1]

"The foregoing evidence clearly indicates the existence of a fixed enzyme potential in all living creatures," Howell

wrote. "This potential ... diminishes in time, subject to the conditions and pace of life."[2]

There was more. Societies with diets rich in enzymes, like the Georgians, Ecuadorians and the Hunzas of northern Pakistan have a high concentration of centurians—people living to more than 100 years of age. These peoples, Howell noted, made "extensive use of fermentation—soy, dairy, vegetables and fruits." Also, they utilized sprouting as well as soaking of seeds, "which increases the enzyme level up to 20 times and raw or undercooked food."[3]

For Howell, it all came down to preserving our enzyme potential.

So can enzyme supplements help us human beings live longer, healthier lives? Perhaps. It's definitely something to think about.

First let's take a look at how systemic enzyme therapy has evolved and is now being investigated around the world for its potential in the treatment of all manner of diseases, from cancer to autism.

BIGGER THAN LIFE

If Howell was the father of food enzymes, the father of systemic enzyme therapy for the treatment of disease was

the equally iconoclastic Max Wolf, whose colorful life and work are chronicled in Lopez, Williams and Miehlke's 1994 book, *Enzymes: The Fountain of Life.*

Wolf was a bigger than life little man at five foot one.

Lopez: "He acted like a magnet to the most beautiful women, the cleverest scientists, the most famous artists and the mightiest politicians. They hung onto his every word and followed his every action."

Actually, he was a bit of a genius.

Wolf was born in Vienna in 1885. An early career as an engineer, with several railway switching patents to his name, gave way to a career as an artist and his rapid ascension to Court Painter to Emperor Franz Joseph of Austria.

Wolf was visiting his brother in New York when the First World War broke out. Rather than return to Vienna, he stayed on in New York and joined his brother in the study of medicine. By his third semester, Lopez notes, he was lecturing at the University, and not long after graduating, he was awarded a full professorship at Fordham. He would be awarded seven different doctorates during the course of his lifetime.

Wolf started out as a gynecologist, running a busy maternity center in a large working class section of Manhattan. But his insatiable mind led him in other

directions as well. He became an ear nose and throat specialist. His interest in hormone secreting glands led him to write one of the first textbooks on endocrinology.

Then he got into genetics.

"Some of his contributions," Lopez notes, "are now used in modern genetic engineering."

But it was Wolf's subsequent interest in enzymes that became his life's passion.

That passion was sparked when Viennese physician Dr. Ernst Freund discovered, in the 1930s, that cancer patients lacked a mysterious substance present in the blood of healthy persons that was capable of destroying cancer cells, thus protecting them by extinguishing cancer in its earliest stages.

Freund named his discovery "normal substance."

During the 1920s and early 1930s, Wolf made frequent trips to Vienna to study with Freund. After Freund's death, he took over this research, and concluded that this "normal substance" had to be an enzyme. In fact, Freund's "normal substance" turned out to be a "hydrolase" enzyme—one which does its work in the presence of water. Further investigation led Wolf to realize that hydrolase enzymes play a key role not only in cancer but in other disease conditions as well.

And so Wolf's life work commenced.

He founded the Biological Research Institute and recruited Dr. Helen Benitez, who had run Columbia University's cell culturing laboratory for years. The two spent the 1950s isolating hydrolase enzymes from all manner of life, purifying these enzymes, and running thousands of laboratory tests to determine which—if any—were capable of destroying cancer cells.

Anything they came up with had to be highly purified and formulated into coated tablets that would make it into the small intestine where they would be broken down and absorbed into the body.

Then there were the safety trials. Huge doses had to be given to animals before they could be administered to humans.

In the end, the team came up with three oral enzyme mixtures, from both animal and plant sources. The first of the Wolf-Benitez enzyme mixtures, as they were called, was designed to deal with inflammatory disorders, like rheumatoid arthritis and coronary artery disease. The next was designed to treat degenerative disorders, like Parkinson's disease and multiple sclerosis. And the third was designed to fight cancer.

Again, in the United States today, these and other enzyme supplements are not designed or approved to diagnose, treat, cure or prevent any disease. There are some exceptions. Certain enzyme-based drugs have been approved by the FDA for medical purposes in hospitals (e.g., TPA).

* * *

Before we go any further, Max Wolf was not the first physician to come up with the idea of treating cancer patients with enzymes. That distinction belongs to the Scottish embryologist John Beard, who wrote in the British journal, *The Lancet,* in 1902, that the pancreatic enzyme trypsin was the body's primary defense against cancer and he believed that it should be used to treat the disease.

Beard was a highly respected scientist. Besides his Ph.D., which covered zoology, physics and botany, he held an advanced doctor of science degree from the University of Manchester. In 1906, he was nominated for the Nobel Prize, in part for work that gave birth to today's theory of the cancer stem cell—the idea that certain cancer cells are responsible for perpetuating the growth of tumors in the

same way that normal stem cells renew and sustain various organs and tissues in our bodies.

It was Beard's work comparing cancer cells to embryo-nurturing cells called trophoblasts, which led to the theory of the cancer stem cell.

Trophoblasts, he found, looked and acted just like cancer cells, multiplying quickly, forming tumor-like masses, even invading nearby tissues. They were just like cancer cells—until they got some kind of signal and settled down and behaved.

Cancer cells, on the other hand, never settle down and behave.

The idea of treating cancer with pancreatic enzymes hit Beard when he discovered that trophoblasts start settling down in the developing embryo the moment the newly formed pancreas starts producing enzymes.

Indeed! If pancreatic enzymes can make these cancer-like trophoblasts settle down, he reasoned, maybe they can make cancer cells settle down and behave too.

It made sense. And so he set to work.

To get the enzymes he needed, he sacrificed newborn lambs, piglets and calves, chopped the pancreas of each into tiny pieces and injected the filtered enzyme-rich juices into the veins or buttocks of his cancer patients.

Sometimes he would inject the enzyme juice directly into tumors.

His treatments weren't always successful, Lopez notes. And the "unpurified juices" sometimes provoked allergic reactions, in several cases sending the patient into shock.

Beard was branded a "mad charlatan" by his colleagues.

But in 1907, he published a book, *The Enzyme Treatment of Cancer and Its Scientific Basis.* In it, he described injecting pancreatic juices into 170 cancer patients, more than half of whom were reportedly helped—their lives were prolonged, some showing no evidence of the tumors that had occupied their bodies.

The book, Lopez notes, created "a furor in England."

And it put a lot of pressure on Beard's colleagues, whose patients were now demanding the miracle juice.

And they got it. The problem was, these doctors ordered their pancreatic juices from pharmacists who got it from the local slaughterhouse. Compared to Beard's freshly squeezed enzyme juices from newborn, newly slaughtered animals, Lopez points out, these juices, "had long since degraded themselves since enzymes are active in aqueous solution and have an active life which can be measured in hours."

Hence, they were inactive by the time they were injected into patients, where they showed no benefit at all.

Just like the pasteurized orange juice at the Lindlahr.

"Dr. Beard's method was quickly forgotten." Lopez wrote.

But the idea of treating cancer patients with enzymes did not go away entirely.

There were sparks of interest in America and elsewhere.[4]

Dr. William Morton of the Post-Graduate Medical School in New York treated 29 cancer patients with the pancreatic enzyme trypsin, with two reported cures and others "progressing favorably," as reported by *The New York Times* in 1906.

Dr. Marshall McDuffie, President of the Homeopathic Medical Society of New York, introduced the use of intravenous injections of trypsin with "encouraging" results.

Dr. Frank LeForest Morse, chair of the gynecology department at the College of Physicians and Surgeons of St. Louis, got a mixed reaction when he stood before his St. Louis Medical Society colleagues in 1934 and reported a 10-percent response rate after a decade of treating cancer patients with injections of pancreatic enzymes.

The Society's medical journal was impressed—some patients reportedly had remission of bone metastases—but the audience from the "Show-Me" state was anything but enthusiastic that day about Morse's crude experiments, accusing him of offering false hope to cancer patients and

implying that the treatment was a cure, which he did not. No further mention of the treatment was made in any of the Society's publications.

The German biochemist Adolph Gaschler reported success treating some cancers by giving patients oral enzymes in 1937.

Then Dr. Wolf came along with the Wolf-Benitez oral formulations in the 1950s, and that's when systemic enzyme therapy took off.

Of course, most countries today require extensive clinical trials, be it a new drug or supplement that may have drug-like qualities, before it can be prescribed freely to patients. This process can take decades. As is usually the case in most scientific advances, more than observational studies are needed. The gold standard usually involves at least one and possibly more double-blind, placebo-controlled, randomized clinical trials.

TALKING PREVENTION

Before he and Ellen Benitez came up with their oral enzyme tablets, Max Wolf had been treating patients with enzyme injections for years. A classical music enthusiast,

he had moved his practice to New York's fashionable Upper East Side and was appointed the official physician for the Metropolitan Opera. Over the years, reportedly, his list of patients came to include the likes of Enrico Caruso and Arturo Toscanini, Marilyn Monroe and Clark Gable, and political heavyweights John Foster Dulles and President John F. Kennedy, known for his persistent back problems.

Most of these patients were treated with injections for inflammatory conditions.

Because of the purity of Wolf's preparations, allergic reactions were usually no longer an issue. But like Beard before him, Wolf was regarded with skepticism and worse by mainstream physicians, even as the Wolf-Benitez enzyme tablets were becoming widely used in Europe.

The cancer formulation, Lopez noted in 1994, "has been administered to about 50,000 cancer patients per year over the past 25 years in western Germany alone."[5] In the same period that the Wolf-Benitez plant- and animal-derived preparations had been available in Europe, more than 20 million prescriptions had been written, with unprescribed use of the over-the-counter digestive preparations even higher.

The use of the Wolf-Benitez enzyme preparations in the treatment of cancer and other conditions, including arthritis, cardiovascular disease, multiple sclerosis, surgical trauma and various injuries, has been investigated in numerous randomized clinical trials internationally.[6]

At the time of Lopez's writing, only 240 cases of side effects had been reported—mostly intestinal gas, or bleeding issues after surgery or an injury. That's far less than 1 percent of the millions and millions of treatments.[7]

Most prescription drugs today have side effects of one sort or another in far more than 1 percent of patients treated.

Why would enzyme supplements be an effective weapon against cancer?

The answer to this question may have to do with the way cancer cells evade the immune system by concealing their identity.

Cancer cells are constantly forming in our bodies. The good news is, these "deranged" cells are usually recognized and eliminated by our immune system. Things get out of hand, Lopez notes, when the deranged cell population gets too high, because of things like environmental pollutants, carcinogens in tobacco smoke, medications that weaken our immune system, poor eating habits, radiation, or

simply the weakening of our body defenses as we age.

Cancer cells begin attaching themselves to cell walls in hidden places and invading tissues. To further escape detection, they cloak themselves in fibrin—the same blood-clotting protein we talked about in the last chapter.

Lopez: "They hide their suspicious markings, their antigens, under a layer of glue so that they are not recognized as enemies."[8]

Protease enzymes dissolve away this fibrin coating.

In fact, when researchers want to test a drug's effectiveness against cancer, one of the things they use are these protein-degrading enzymes to dissolve away the fibrin coat first, exposing the cancer cell's surface antigens to the drug.[9]

It follows that enzymes can strip away fibrin from cancer cells in the body in this same way, making them more identifiable to the immune system.

Enzymes also stimulate macrophages to release TNF (tumor necrosis factor), a powerful killer of cancer cells. Austrian in vitro studies have borne this out, using protease enzymes bromelain and papain from the pineapple and the papaya, and this strategy has been used successfully in the treatment of cancers.[10]

Another strategy cancer cells use to evade the immune system is shedding identifying antigens from their surfaces, just as military aircraft release drones to act as decoys, to distract enemy radar and draw fire.

These decoy antigens draw the attention of the immune system. Antibodies attach to them, forming immune complexes, rather than going after the fibrin-coated cancer cells.

Too many immune complexes can actually "inhibit the activity of macrophages," according to Lopez. "Their ability to devour and destroy is lost."[11]

Enzymes go after these decoy immune complexes.

All this has led physicians in Europe and other parts of the world, including Japan, India, Russia and Australia, to add enzymes to radiation and chemotherapy.

Besides helping shrink tumors, researchers report that the addition of enzyme supplements can reduce the side effects from radiation and chemotherapy, as well as making it possible to use less radiation and chemotherapy and get the same therapeutic effect.[12]

Lopez says, "A significant number of oncologists in Germany, Italy and France already use enzymes for their cancer patients in the hospital."[13]

How long, he wonders, will it take for American researchers to take enzymes seriously and catch up to the rest of the world?

At the time of his writing, in 1993, the only enzyme approved in the United States for the treatment of cancer was L-asparaginase, for acute lymphocytic leukemia. Twenty years later, in response to an inquiry by the authors of this book, the National Cancer Institute reported that the only enzyme it is currently funding for clinical trials is L-asparaginase, for acute lymphocytic leukemia.

It isn't just about cancer. The National Center for Complementary and at the National Institutes of Health is currently funding no clinical trials involving enzyme preparations—plant or animal.

Lopez: "Can American medicine ignore a treatment modality that is at present prescribed legally, ethically and reportedly with great success to over 200,000 patients per year," he wrote in 1993, "including 70,000 cancer patients and 50,000 patients with vascular disorders. A treatment that has been administered to over 15 million patients during the past 15 years and which by all reports appears to be safer than most other modalities of treatment currently available for the same conditions?"[14]

The European scientists, he notes, believe that people can actually cut their risk of developing cancer by taking enzyme supplements.

We're talking prevention. So there's a lot at stake here. And it's not just about cancer.

ABOUT CARDIOVASCULAR DISEASE

The leading cause of death in the United States, just above cancer, is cardiovascular disease. This includes all the diseases of the heart and the blood vessels throughout the body. The most common form of cardiovascular disease is atherosclerosis, which involves narrowing of the artery walls with the accumulation of plaque.

It starts when the delicate lining of the artery walls becomes damaged by smoking, high cholesterol, high blood pressure, diabetes, etc., and circulating "bad" cholesterol starts to accumulate inside the artery walls. White blood cells arriving to break down the cholesterol become part of the toxic mess, and the formation of plaque. Add to this circulating immune complexes settling inside artery walls, along with accumulating fibrin, and you've got the perfect recipe for inflammation, with an

increasing risk of life-threatening blood clots forming, blocking circulation to the heart, the brain and the lungs.

There was no doubt in Howell's mind that a big contributor to this inflammatory cascade is incomplete digestion due to the absence of food enzymes in the cooked and processed foods we eat.

This is where he saw the aforementioned whales and native Eskimos going one up on us, with their enzyme-rich, high-fat raw diets, and their clean arteries.

Then there's the aforementioned decline in our enzyme production as we age, and its effect on the health of our arteries.

In 1962, the renowned British pathologist, Dr. C. W. M. Abrams reported his studies showing that the enzyme activity in the walls of our blood vessels becomes "progressively" weaker as we age, and as atherosclerosis develops and becomes more "severe."[15]

The same has been found true of man's best friend, whose cooked and processed K-9 diet has brought the same inflammatory cascade to his arteries. And the more advanced the dog's atherosclerosis, the lower its enzyme levels.[16]

So we need enzymes working in our blood vessels at all times. Enzymes are critical to their maintenance.

And supplemental enzymes may help prevent this inflammatory cascade, by working with your body's own natural mechanisms.

Recent studies by researchers in England, Spain, Austria and the Far East suggest that enzyme supplements may be effective in relieving chest pains (angina) and restoring normal blood flow to narrowed coronary arteries, as well as helping people with disorders of the veins. These include: phlebitis, which is inflammation of the veins in the legs, due to blood clots; deep vein thrombosis (DVT), blood clots that form in the veins of the legs and can travel up into the lungs; and post-thrombotic syndrome, where blood clots in the legs leave people with long-term pain, heaviness and swelling in their legs, as well as varicose veins and leg ulcers.

These symptoms become more common as we age.

In the case of phlebitis and post-phlebitis syndrome, the Spanish researchers armed with enzyme supplements relieved patient symptoms in just weeks, compared to conventional therapies, which took months to work.[17]

Deep vein thrombosis, which strikes 2 million Americans every year, killing approximately 200,000, may be prevented or at least reduced by enzyme supplements. That's what British researchers concluded when they gave plant-derived

enzyme supplements to people at high risk for these blood clots before they boarded long airplane flights. Nobody in the enzyme group developed blood clots, while five of 92 people on placebo capsules developed DVTs. At the time of this writing, the FDA has not evaluated this enzyme formulation for the prevention of deep vein thrombosis.[18]

The more we look at the science, however, the more we recognize the importance of enzymes in our daily health and overall well-being, the consequences of an enzyme-deficient diet, and how supplemental enzymes along with other factors may help play a role in reducing our risk of developing these inflammatory diseases by cutting inflammation off at the pass.

The same is true for arthritis.

Of course, legally it is necessary and prudent to again remind readers and state: **Supplements, just like medications or drugs, can have side effects and interact with other medications or foods.** As such, there is a standard disclaimer for virtually all supplements in the United States that reads something like this: "These statements have not been evaluated by the Food and Drug Administration (FDA). Supplements as defined by the FDA are not intended to diagnose, treat, cure or prevent any disease." And: "Always check with your own physician

or healthcare professional before taking any supplements or medications."

TIME TO HEAL

When it came to arthritis, Howell was thinking enzymes from the beginning.

Why? Because in his mind, arthritis also has roots in inflammation resulting from incomplete digestion. This is why, he reasoned, arthritic symptoms improve during fasting periods—because the digestive system gets the day off and the immune system can devote all of its forces to dealing with inflammatory problems in the joints, instead of having to help out with digestion.

And with fasting comes a break in the flow of undigested food antigens and a reduction in the flow of inflammation-breeding immune complexes and bacterial toxins finding their way through the sea of extracellular fluids into the synovial joints.

The whole body gets the day off from inflammation, and time to heal.

The first to connect incomplete protein digestion with rheumatoid arthritis was British researcher Dr. Arnold

Renshaw. When his patients took human digestive enzyme capsules with their meals, their arthritis reportedly improved—not just rheumatoid arthritis, but patients with osteoarthritis and severe spondylitis, or inflammation of the spine, who had failed all other treatments.[19]

Howell reported similar results with his own enzyme mixture, derived from the aspergillus fungus. He had his patients empty two to five capsules onto their food. Worst cases of long-standing osteoarthritis and rheumatoid arthritis reportedly came around. Slow responders, he noted, could be speeded up by increasing the number of capsules they were taking.

He liked to tell the story of his 80-year-old bedridden grandmother who suffered from heart disease, asthma, arthritis and kidney disorder.

"Within several weeks of the inauguration of the supplementation program," he wrote, "she was doing all the house chores for a family of four—cooking, laundry, cleaning, as well as readying, praying, watching television and socialization. From bed to full activity; this high energy continued for over 2 years."

Of course, these were not double-blind, clinically proven studies; they were observational and anecdotal. Nevertheless, they did support the concepts that Howell

and others purported. Frequently in medicine, it's simple observation that leads to great discoveries.

The bottom line for Howell: "A human is nourished and maintained not by what he eats, but by what is digested."[20] And while the authors believe you are what you eat, we believe even more that you are what you are able to digest and absorb. Lopez co-author, Dr. Klaus Miehlke, an internationally recognized expert in systemic enzyme therapy and professor of rheumatology at the University of Mainz, in Germany, found enzyme mixtures "as good as, or superior to, other anti-rheumatic agents on account of their comparable efficacy and their lack of dangerous side effects."[21]

Researchers doing studies in Germany, Austria, Pakistan and India, report that the plant enzyme bromelain, from the pineapple, combined with the human pancreatic enzyme trypsin, in a coated tablet, work as well as conventional anti-inflammatory drugs in arthritis, but without some of the side effects.[22]

It makes sense, because rheumatoid arthritis patients have been shown to have elevated levels of immune complexes in their blood, and in their joint capsules. And just like cancer cells, Lopez notes, these immune complexes become cloaked in a fibrin "mantle," which hides them from the immune system.

Enzyme supplements strip away the fibrin cloaking the immune complexes in the joints, rendering them identifiable to the immune forces.

Suddenly it's open season, and the hunt is on.

And as immune complexes are eliminated, inflammation settles down and joints have a chance to heal.

So why aren't enzyme preparations being studied to this extent in America?

Again, a lot of it has to do with economics. It costs a pharmaceutical company approximately 1 billion dollars to develop a new drug and put it through years of clinical trials to get FDA approval. All too often, a drug doesn't pan out, which puts even more pressure on drugs that do get approved to make the money back.

After approval, the pharmaceutical company has 17 years to sell its new drug before its patent runs out and other manufacturers are free to make and sell their own "bioequivalent" versions of it—a generic version.

Natural products, like enzymes, come directly from Nature, so there's no new molecule to patent. Efforts are now being made through genetic engineering to create patent-possible enzyme products. Until this happens, pharmaceutical companies are unlikely to invest a lot of money putting enzyme mixtures through

FDA trials with no patent on the other end to protect their investments.

And while doctors are free to give a patient any natural product they choose, there are factors working against them doing this. One is that mainstream medicine is reluctant to change the way it thinks.

Doctors like to prescribe medications that have been deemed "safe and effective" by the FDA. And for good reason. In our litigious society, there's the risk of being sued for not giving the patient the prescription drug, or recommending a supplement that the doctor is not familiar with, or one that has not had the documented research in the United States that would be approved by the FDA.

There's a lot of pressure on doctors from pharmaceutical manufacturers to prescribe their products.

That's why, in many minds, more research is not being done with enzymes in America, and why mainstream medicine isn't using enzymes more often, even when the European evidence is compelling, as in the case of injuries. The "Catch 22" is that more placebo-controlled clinical studies are needed or must be done in the United States for American physicians to generally consider recommending supplemental enzymes.

THE HEALING PROCESS

Whenever an injury occurs, whether it's a finger pierced by a sewing needle, multiple contusions resulting from an automobile accident, or a sports sprain, a successful healing depends to a great extent on the availability of the body's enzyme forces. The same is true of local infections.

There's a paradox here, in that when supplemental enzymes are used to treat injuries and infections, as they are in Europe and other parts of the world, they are often referred to as anti-inflammatory enzymes. It makes sense. With an acute injury or an infection, where the area is all swollen and red, and painful, the whole idea should be to bring down inflammation, right?

Actually, as Lopez notes, the opposite is true.

Inflammation is not a disease. Rather, he points out, it's a sign that healing and repair are taking place. Blood vessels in the affected area have to be dilated and made permeable to admit as many macrophages and other troops as needed into the area to attack any pathogens—viral, bacterial, etc.—that might be involved. Once this is accomplished, the area has to be cleared of any toxins, as well as dead tissue, followed by the repair and rebuilding of the damaged structures.

Enzymes are involved in this healing process every step of the way, and studies have shown that enzyme supplements may speed this healing process.

German karate fighters taking protease enzyme supplements, combining pineapple-derived bromelain and papain from the papaya with pancreatic enzymes, before matches saw their bruises disappear in just 7 days, compared to 16 days for fighters taking placebo capsules, with full movement restored in just 5 days compared to 12 days and longer for the placebo group.[23]

Physicians treating other athletes, including German Olympic athletes, using similar plant/animal derived enzyme combinations, saw all manner of sports injuries—contusions, joint and ligament ruptures, torn muscles, vertebral injuries, knee injuries, etc.—heal dramatically faster on three to six enzyme capsules a day.[24]

According to the Enzyme Research Institute, founded by Max Wolf, "scarcely an international sporting event takes place without some of the active participants using enzyme preparations. This applies to world championships in soccer, handball and ice hockey, and the rather brutal American football, all sports where the risks of injury to the participants are high."[25]

Enzymes are being used to treat everyday injuries worldwide.

In some countries they are also being used to reduce healing and hospital time for people undergoing surgery, as long as the patient doesn't have a bleeding condition.

According to the Enzyme Research Institute, "At present, operations are being undertaken in a number of European centers where the full range of enzyme action is exploited both before and after the surgical intervention."[26]

And now there's autism.

HEALING AN AMERICAN EPIDEMIC

At the time of this writing, one in every 88 American children is being born on the autism spectrum. What was first described in the 1940s has now reached epidemic proportions, with little in the way of medicinal help for children whose socialization skills have been so severely affected by this disabling neurologic disorder.

And yet, two recent American studies suggest that enzymes may help.

One such study, headed by leading autism researcher Dr. Mark A. Brudnak, Ph.D., N.D., in 2003, was based

on the observation that children with autism have difficulty digesting proteins from wheat and dairy foods.[27]

Many also suffer from leaky gut syndrome. Partially digested proteins, called exorphins, cross the intestinal wall, entering the bloodstream and make their way to the brain, where they have a narcotic-like effect, disrupting brain function.

In this study, the researchers went after these exorphins with a specially designed digestive enzyme formulation that included pineapple-derived bromelain, as well as other protein-degrading enzymes, and plant-derived phytase, which helps digest grains and seeds, liberating all-important phosphorous, along with essential minerals calcium, magnesium, iron and zinc.

For 12 weeks, the children took their enzyme capsule with each meal. They were evaluated for improvement in everything affected by autism, from eye contact, socialization and attention, to hyperactivity, anxiety, comprehension, speech, digestion and sleep.

The researchers reported "an overwhelmingly positive trend ... for each of the parameters." The two greatest improvements were in socialization and hyperactivity, with 90 percent and 80 percent improvement, respectively.

For many, it was like night and day.

And there were "very few" negative reactions.

In December 2011, researchers at Ohio State University announced the results of a multi-center study using a digestive enzyme formulation called CM-AT to relieve the gastrointestinal problems suffered by children with autism spectrum disorders.[28]

In this case, they were acting on the observation by Dr. Joan Fallon in San Francisco that when gastrointestinal function is helped, autism behavioral symptoms also improve.

This was a double-blind, placebo-controlled trial, at 15 centers nationally, with neither the doctors nor the parents or children knowing who was getting the enzymes and who was getting the placebo capsules. Though the results have not yet been fully published, it was announced that the study met both its primary and secondary goals—improvement in digestion and improvement in the behavioral issues that plague children with autism.

The results were so impressive that the researchers went right into a second study at 19 centers across the United States, with the FDA placing CM-AT on a special "Fast Track" program reserved to expedite approval of promising new drugs for serious or fatal conditions.[29]

This time, it appears that enzymes may come to the rescue for children with autism.

The list goes on—enzymes in the treatment of allergies and migraine headaches, enzymes in the treatment of multiple sclerosis, enzymes for shingles, etc.

There virtually isn't a disease on this planet that hasn't been treated with enzymes, with or without the assistance of medicine. Enzymes are, after all, Nature's workers. They are our body's keepers, and they are on duty 24/7, digesting what we eat, maintaining and rebuilding systems, providing the spark of life for every body function, for every breath we take, helping keep our blood vessels and joints clean and in good working order, and assisting the immune system in ridding the body of foreign invaders and toxins.

Given the evidence, there is good reason to believe that the use of digestion enzyme supplements may indeed improve the overall quality of our health and lives, by doing the job of the food enzymes missing from our diet, by giving the overworked pancreas a break and keeping it in good health for the long haul, and by facilitating more complete digestion—particularly that of cooked meat.

More complete digestion alone, it appears, may reduce the ongoing inflammatory cascade that is behind the

aforementioned degenerative diseases, thereby reducing our risk for developing these diseases.

An NEC pilot study conducted at Logan University supported Dr. Kouchakoff's findings concerning cooked and processed foods and leukocytosis, and more. In this double-blind, placebo-controlled study 10 healthy volunteers ate a meal consisting of chili, cheese, and crackers. Five of the study participants received two digestive enzyme capsules, which they took just prior to eating, while the other five received two placebo capsules. Blood was drawn from all 10 participants immediately prior to and 45 minutes after they began their meal. Their blood was analyzed to measure increases in an array of inflammatory markers, including white blood cells (lymphocytes, monocytes and granulocytes), interleukin 6 (an inflammatory protein in the body), and C-Reactive protein, which is also involved in inflammation.

On average, although not statistically significant, all measurable markers of inflammation were attenuated as a result of taking digestive enzymes along with the test meal. There were important trends with those taking the digestive enzymes, suggesting that various measures of inflammation may be reduced by taking the enzyme

supplements prior to the meal. Future larger studies are planned to further investigate this. The possibility of reducing one's inflammation "load" could have tremendous health benefits!

At the time of the writing of this book, a larger double-blind study is currently underway to further confirm the ability of supplemental digestive enzymes to reduce the inflammatory cascade that comes with eating a cooked meal.

We're not just talking about preventing cancer, heart disease and arthritis, although anything that reduces these risks is worth its weight in gold. This is about quality of life. Anything that reduces excess inflammation is going to improve the overall quality of our lives.

Howell saw it from the beginning.

"If you take in outside enzyme reinforcements for predigestion," he wrote, "The Law of Adaptive Secretion of Digestive Enzymes and your own food enzyme stomach will become your best friends. ... Good enzyme nutrition needs outside enzyme reinforcements. Don't disappoint Nature—give her the outside enzyme reinforcements your primordial ancestors had been getting for millions of years."[30]

Lopez extends the benefit to better all-around digestion: "Better absorption of essential vitamins, minerals, trace elements, fatty acids and nutrients

translates into a better supply, and thus into a more efficient and healthier body."[31]

So can enzyme supplements really help us live longer?

If adding digestive enzyme supplements to our daily diet—along with a healthy diet and exercise and not smoking—provides more complete digestion and reduces inflammation and our risk of developing cancer and heart disease alone, then the answer to that question would be yes—theoretically.

In the next and final chapter we'll look at how we can bring the power of enzymes back into our lives.

CHAPTER 7

BRINGING THE LIFE ELEMENT BACK INTO YOUR LIFE

For Doc Howell, enzyme supplements were the missing link in human nutrition. They were the means of replacing the food enzymes cooked, pasteurized and processed out of the foods we eat. They were the key to better health and a longer life through more complete digestion.

That's what he believed.

But not just any enzyme supplements. Howell was talking about enzyme supplements that do their work in what he called the food enzyme stomach, as Nature intended.

Until now, the vast majority of supplements used in systemic enzyme therapy have been animal-derived, coated pancreatic enzyme capsules or tablets designed to dissolve and do their work in the small intestine.

These are not food enzyme supplements per se.

The majority of their work is not done in the food enzyme stomach.

They contribute little or nothing to predigestion.

And this is where enzyme therapy has fallen short.

There is, however, another approach to systemic enzyme therapy growing nationally that does work in Nature's intended way. What's different about this approach? It uses plant-derived enzyme supplements, which do their work in the food enzyme stomach. It's all about predigestion. And it's pure Howell. The approach involves using food enzyme supplements to achieve more complete digestion and deliver the nutrition needed that may support the ailing body system to heal itself. It's all about maintaining homeostasis, and whatever healing takes place flows from that.

And it's not just about disease.

For Doc Howell and others, the theory behind this approach has to do with maintaining and ensuring overall good health—not just catching a disease before it cripples or kills us, but preventing it from developing in the first place. How? Through more complete digestion, our body may be able to reduce the inflammatory cascade that leads to the development of degenerative diseases like rheumatoid arthritis, diabetes, heart disease and cancer.

And preserve our "enzyme potential" as we age.

It's all about living healthier, hopefully longer lives, the way Nature originally intended.

All things being equal, many experts agree that a combination of eating fresh, enzyme-rich foods, portion control, exercise, the use of enzyme supplements, and no smoking is the best way to support and maintain good health. Taking into account that enzyme-rich foods are not what they used to be back in Doc Howell's day puts more importance now on the potential value of food enzyme supplements to achieve more complete digestion, and to preserve our enzyme potential as we age.

Let's start with the foods.

GOOD SOURCES OF FOOD ENZYMES

Two basic criteria govern enzymes in foods.

The first has to do with caloric content. The higher a food's calorie content, the more enzymes it will contain. Hence, a pound of avocado will contain more enzymes than a pound of lettuce. High enzyme foods can include bananas, avocados, grapes, mangoes, pineapple, olives, fresh or raw dates and figs, raw honey, milk and butter.

The second criteria has to do with the *type* of food it is. The avocado, which is high in fat, is going to be high in lipase—the fat-digesting enzyme. High-starch foods, like potatoes, contain a lot of amylase, and high-protein foods contain proteases, like cathepsin in meats.

The intended purpose of these enzymes is to serve the digestive and metabolic needs of their original owner during life and to assist in the cellular breakdown of that organism after death. However, when that organism becomes food, its enzymes function as digestive enzymes for the new owner. Such is the case with cathepsin, or papain from the papaya, or bromelain from the pineapple. All three function as protein-digesting enzymes.

They also make excellent meat tenderizers.

Other sources of protease enzymes include eggs, natural cheeses, ginger, kiwi fruit, soy, wheat, barley, bulgur and wild rice. While some still advocate the use of raw milk fasting for therapeutic purposes, and steak tartare remains a delicacy served in select restaurants. Medical experts agree that neither raw milk nor uncooked meat should be consumed as a regular source of nutrition. Bacterial contamination is a serious concern, among other issues.

Again, what we've learned about enzymes is that foods high in fat-digesting lipase include avocados and olives, as well as bananas, cherries, figs and grapes.

Foods rich in carbohydrases, which digest carbohydrates, include raw honey, sweet potato and wheat.

Finally, foods rich in cellulase, which converts cellulose into energy-providing glucose, include vegetables and grains, like wheat and millet, and high-fiber fruits, like apples, papayas and pears. The human body does not make its own cellulase, so this enzyme must come from outside food sources.

Like everything else in life, moderation is key. Simply eating avocados all day is not the answer. We all need to maintain a balanced diet.

Dr. Howard Loomis makes a good point about digesting cellulose. In his book, *Enzymes: A Key to Health,* Dr. Loomis notes that most vegetables are covered with a thin film of cellulose, which gets in the way of our digesting them. This is why a lot of people complain of intestinal gas when they eat raw vegetables. One way of getting rid of this layer of cellulose is by more thoroughly chewing raw vegetables when we eat them. This will break down the cellulose layer and release the cellulase enzymes to aid in digestion.

"People who claim they cannot eat raw food because of discomfort from intestinal gas, are really saying they do not chew raw food thoroughly," Dr. Loomis concludes.[1] But we do know that there are enzyme supplements available that can support healthy digestion of raw vegetables.

Remember Doc Howell's bottom line: Substitute raw for cooked "as much as possible."

Again, these foods include bananas, avocados, grapes, mangoes, olives, fresh or raw dates and figs, raw honey, and other natural foods moderately high in food enzymes.

A diet containing 75-percent raw calories and 25-percent cooked calories, Howell wrote, "is a vast improvement over the virtually enzyme-less diet used by most people."[2]

And there's an added bonus to eating raw. Raw foods are less fattening than cooked foods. Besides not contributing food enzymes to aid in the digestive process, Howell and others believed that cooked foods can, in a way, overstimulate the endocrine system, which leads to weight gain.

In fact, farmers looking to fatten up their pigs years ago learned they could do so by switching from raw to cooked potatoes.

So there's a lot to be said for eating more fresh raw foods, such as fruits and vegetables.

In recent years, starch blockers have become quite the craze in America. Marketed as weight-loss miracles, these starch-blocking supplements are nothing more than enzyme inhibitors that are designed to block the digestion of starches, so they will pass through the body unabsorbed.

Researchers are concerned about the long-term effects of starch blockers. Short-term effects can include fermentation of undigested starches as they accumulate in the colon, producing gas, and causing bloating and diarrhea.[3]

Finally, there's the question about the enzyme content of today's fruits and vegetables. While the shelf life of produce has increased exponentially with new technologies, this benefit has unfortunately come at the cost of enzyme potential.

A look at milk, once Nature's most curative elixir, tells the story.

A MILK MAID'S TALE

Raw milk is probably the last thing a doctor would think of prescribing today, and for good reason—because of the very real danger of bacterial contamination. But back in 1905, when Dr. Charles Sanford Porter published the first

edition of his book, *Milk Diet as a Remedy for Chronic Disease*, detailing his 41 years of treating more than 18,000 patients, he placed himself in a historical context that dated back to the time of Hippocrates, the Father of Medicine.

Man's cultivation of raw milk from domesticated animals began 6,000 years ago, in Neolithic Britain. That's when the milking began. And it's a historical fact that the Father of Medicine himself prescribed raw milk as a cure for tuberculosis, then known as phthisis, the Greek word for consumption, which he was the first to identify in 400 B.C.[4]

By 1905, the "raw milk diet," or fast, was an accepted remedy for a wide range of illnesses back then. The Porter regimen—a milk only diet—called for an average six quarts of raw milk daily for a minimum of four weeks, which Porter found to be sufficient for a variety of diseases. These afflictions included, in the medical vernacular of the day, *nervous prostration* (irritable weakness and depression), psoriasis and other skin disorders, anemia, *catarrh* (inflammation of the mucous membranes), indigestion, constipation, *biliousness* (excessive secretion of bile), hay fever, insomnia, stomach ulcers, malaria, rheumatism, and more.[5]

What is it about raw milk that is thought to be so healthful?

For one thing, it possesses all of the eight essential amino acids, which our bodies do not manufacture, but which are important to help develop protein.

Then there's immune-stimulating lactoferrin, a protein that improves our absorption and assimilation of iron, as well as having antioxidant and possibly anticancer properties. Lactoferrin has shown properties that may aid in reducing symptoms of stomach and intestinal ulcers, and hepatitis C. It also has properties shown to help fight bacterial and viral infections. Immunoglobulins in milk are also active against an array of viruses, bacteria and bacterial toxins.

Raw milk is rich in vitamins A, K, E, and C, and the B-complex vitamins, as well essential minerals, including calcium and phosphorus. In addition, raw milk contains beneficial bacteria, which aid in digestion, and cholesterol, which is essential for the building and maintenance of healthy cell walls. All this is but a sampling of why milk has been referred to as the "complete food."[6]

Last, but by no means least, there are some 60 enzymes present in raw milk, including amylase, bacteria-produced lactase, lipases, phosphatases, and milk's chief protease

enzyme, plasmin, all of which take a big load off the pancreas to produce digestive enzymes. Good protein digestion reduces the inflammatory food antigens and bacterial toxins that we talked about in Chapter Five.

In addition, plasmin releases amino acids that are beneficial to our immune system, including glutamine, which is the major fuel for our disease-fighting white blood cells. Glutamine has also been reported to help reduce leaky gut syndrome by tightening up junctions in the intestinal lining.

Lysozyme, like lactoferrin, also kills off a lot of bad bacteria, tipping the scales in favor of the good bacteria in our digestive tract.

We could go on. Suffice it to say, raw milk has a wide range of therapeutic benefits, owing in large part to its working army of enzymes.

Again, drinking raw milk is not recommended today, because of the high risk of contamination. But back when families had cows grazing in the backyard and at local dairies, if someone went on a fresh, raw milk fast, it was hypothesized that they would be getting all the essential nutrients they needed to maintain life, while their pancreas would be getting a much needed rest thanks to the food enzymes contained in the milk. The belief was

that more complete digestion meant reduced inflammation, while the fully fueled immune system and the body's metabolic enzymes would be able to concentrate their resources fighting off disease, and repairing and rebuilding damaged and diseased organs and tissues.

The milk fast made perfect sense to Doc Howell and others, as the science emerged.

It was like going on a fast without really fasting.

But the milk fast wouldn't be worth anything without the enzymes.

And these precious food enzymes were the first to go when milk production became industrialized and pasteurization took over. Other nutritious elements suffered as well.

Pasteurization was inevitable, because with milk no longer making its way directly from the family cow or the local dairy to the family table, contamination was inevitable. The keeping of the cows in large sheds, sometimes underground, the unsanitary handling and storing of the milk, the lack of refrigeration, all contributed to widespread contamination and disease, including tuberculosis.

Pasteurization also brought increased shelf life. Today, a quart of milk is frequently good weeks after the "sell by" date has passed.

The first law requiring commercial milk to be pasteurized was in Chicago, in 1908. Essentially, a major source of food enzymes disappeared overnight, as did the raw "milk cure," which reportedly served as a remedy for so many chronic diseases for centuries, though it has survived to this day on a very limited basis. Again, raw milk is not without significant risks, and the authors are not recommending it.

One could say, with a degree of irony, that pasteurization was the mother of modern enzyme therapy. Pasteurization forced Howell and others to look elsewhere for the mysterious life element that was suddenly missing from Nature's elixirs. It led them to enzyme supplements.

And now produce is heading the way of milk.

LIFE VS. SHELF LIFE

It's all about extending shelf life. Efforts include the aforementioned use of refrigerated warehouses with controlled humidity and the removal of ethylene gas, all to prevent enzymes in the fruits and vegetables from becoming active. As a result, the shelf life of produce has been extended from days to months. Now, with TILLING,

where genetic changes are chemically induced to knock out the ripening gene, and with it the ripening enzymes, industry appears to be on the way to further reducing food enzyme activity.[7]

The fact is, many of today's fresh fruits and vegetables are no longer as rich a source of active food enzymes as they were in Doc Howell's day.

Nobody's breeding the vitamins and minerals out of produce, just the enzyme activity.

Canned fruits and vegetables have little or no enzyme content, nor do factory-produced fruit juices, which have had the enzymes pasteurized and processed out of them.[8] Intentional? Of course not. It just happened. But some scientists now believe that food enzyme supplements are even more important as a means of achieving complete digestion and delivering vitamins and minerals to our cells.

ABOUT FOOD ENZYME SUPPLEMENTS

Food enzyme supplements have come a long way since Jokichi Takamine was awarded the first microbial enzyme patent for Takadiastase, in 1894. Takadiastase was labelled as an amylase because starch was thought to be the cause

of dyspepsia, or upset stomach. But there were other digestive enzymes in there as well, with a whole lot of "side activity" going on as a result.

And the formulation varied somewhat from batch to batch.

Today it's all about purity and consistency. Food enzyme supplements sold nationally are highly observed and scrutinized by the FDA as food additives and/or dietary supplements under GMP (Good Manufacturing Practices) guidelines to insure quality, purity and safety, and consistency from one lot to the next.

The most common source of food enzymes for digestive supplements is the fungus aspergillus, which is grown on various food materials, such as wheat bran or soybeans. Different combinations of these growth mediums, or substrates, produce different enzymes. Enzymes grown on high-protein food materials, like soybeans, will produce proteases; those grown on high-starch foods, like corn or rice, will produce amylase. Extracts from the enzymes produced are then purified and dried into powders, combined to achieve the desired formulation and then put into capsules.

Bacteria are also a good source of enzymes. And a lot of proteases come from plants, like papayas and pineapples.

So what should you look for in a good digestive enzyme supplement?

Lipase is probably the first thing to look for, because there are a number of people who are lipase deficient, and complete digestion of fats is very important.

Next is protease, because the amino acids released when proteins are broken down are the most important signaling molecules in our body. We need the protease to break down proteins into amino acids, and to digest those "burnt red meats" we're so fond of, which can cause so much trouble if they're not completely digested.

Of the carbohydrases, lactase is the most important for the millions who are lactose intolerant. But a variety of carbohydrases is good to have in a digestive supplement.

Then there's cellulase, which breaks down fiber, and which our bodies do not produce. This enzyme comes from the foods we eat or supplements. How important cellulase is in supplements varies from person to person.

Capsules should be swallowed at the beginning of a meal.

Any way you do it, Howell wrote, "You are replacing enzymes which are supposed to be in your food, but are not."

That's the bottom line, and it's a good thing.

While they are very safe, a very small percentage of people may have an allergic reaction to digestive enzyme

supplements, with symptoms typical of any other food allergy. Other people may take a few days for the bacteria and other microorganisms living in their digestive systems to adjust to enzyme supplements. Any resulting gas, bloating and irregularity usually should disappear after a few days.

If someone has problems with digestive enzymes, they should stop taking them and check with their healthcare professional.

Now comes the big question: Why should we consider food enzyme supplements, especially if we're healthy?

Maybe, like Dr. Howell said, it's because we're not really as healthy as we appear to be.

Let's start with digestive problems.

DIGESTIVE PROBLEMS: AM I AT RISK?

Recalling the 1988 Surgeon General's Report on Nutrition and Health, digestive problems added up to the number one health problem in the United States. According to the American Gastroenterological Association, 50 percent of all Americans—more than 150 million—are affected by some form of digestive problems.[9] Studies indicate that 25 million American adults suffer

daily from esophageal reflux disease, a condition causing stomach acid to back up into the esophagus, causing heartburn and sometimes regurgitation. A total of 60 million suffer from "acid reflux" at least once each month.

As many as 38 percent of all adults in the Western World suffer from recurring symptoms of indigestion, including chronic, recurring pain, abdominal fullness, bloating, belching, nausea and heartburn. And 11 percent of adults worldwide suffer from irritable bowel syndrome, with symptoms ranging from chronic pain and bloating to alternating constipation and diarrhea.[10]

In a 2013 pharmaceutical industry survey, 72 percent of 2,000 adults said they experience at least one of the following symptoms multiple times a month: diarrhea, gas, bloating, stomach pain, frequent bowel movements, unexplained weight loss and non-specific gastrointestinal discomfort.[11]

Not one of us is a stranger to digestive problems.

One has only to look at the billions of dollars being spent each year on antacids to see how widespread digestive problems are. And yet, antacids and proton pump inhibitors—drugs that block or reduce hydrochloric acid production—are not always appropriate for gastrointestinal problems. Why? Because the problem may have nothing

to do with acid, and we need hydrochloric acid in our stomach to activate pepsin for protein digestion.

Shutting down acid production may block the first stage of protein digestion. This may put extra stress on the pancreas. From there, if there is extra stress, it can cause things to go downhill. As we've seen, with immune cells responding to assist in protein digestion and to clean up the toxic mess resulting from bad bacterial overgrowth and the release of bacterial toxins, all of which may lead to leaky bowel syndrome and a host of degenerative diseases.

The last thing you want to do is block acid production if you don't have to.

The time to use acid-blocking drugs, according to many physicians today, is primarily when the mucosal lining of the stomach has become compromised, possibly from emotional stress or other causes, resulting in heartburn. It's a good idea to give the cells that make up the mucosal lining a break from acid exposure and a chance to recover and start producing adequate mucus again. Proton pump inhibitors are means of doing this. But many scientists believe that they should only be used long enough to restore the mucosal lining.

In many cases, more complete digestion may help reduce digestive problems.

So we're back to predigestion, and this is where supplemental enzymes come in.

Supplemental food enzymes, as we've seen, can function as replacements for food enzymes that are being cooked, pasteurized, processed and bred out of the foods we eat.

Adding food enzyme supplements to our diet, Dr. Loomis writes, puts the food enzyme stomach back to work, to the degree that it is again capable of digesting up to 60 percent of the foods we consume.[12]

It doesn't stop there. In the Northwestern University study cited earlier in this book, amylase supplements not only digested starches alongside salivary amylase in the food enzyme stomach, 51 percent of the supplemental amylase survived the acidity of the lower stomach and went on to perform double duty, working alongside pancreatic enzymes in the small intestine.[13]

All of this may help take a big strain off the pancreas and make for a healthier digestive system.

It's important to reinforce here that digestive enzyme supplements are not drugs. They are not intended to diagnose, treat, cure, or prevent any disease. But they may help support your body's own natural mechanisms of digestion, and in doing so, they may help facilitate more complete digestion and support digestive health.

That's where the evidence is pointing.

Recent studies have shown that food enzyme supplements can help relieve gastrointestinal problems by working with your body's own natural mechanisms of digestion. This includes symptoms caused by lactose intolerance, as well as the relief of intestinal gas, bloating and diarrhea that can come following a meal of fermentable carbohydrates—i.e., beans.[14]

Then there's hard-to-digest gluten, which has become something of a national obsession, to the point that manufacturers are going to great lengths and expense to produce gluten-free wheat products. Laboratory and animal studies have shown that food enzyme supplements are effective in breaking down gluten and may offer hope to millions suffering from gluten intolerance.[15]

The ability of food enzyme supplements to help relieve digestive symptoms is the reason why patients and their physicians came to Howell when he first started using them in his own practice.

So that's one good reason to take them—not just when problems occur, but to help support and maintain healthy digestion.

Again, unlike pancreatic enzymes, food enzymes supplements work in the enzyme stomach, with

predigestion translating into more complete digestion all the way downstream. This brings us to nutrition.

GOOD NUTRITION MATTERS

We all need our nutrients. And when we don't get them from the foods we eat, there are consequences.

A diet deficient in protein can cause fatigue, shrinkage of muscle tissue, loss of appetite, and edema, or a build-up of fluids, especially in the feet and ankles. Protein deficiency can also cause slow growth in children.

Symptoms of carbohydrate deficiency include fatigue, irritability, loss of muscle mass, diarrhea or constipation and frequent headaches. A carbohydrate-deficient diet when taken to extremes, also forces our body to break down protein to maintain blood sugar levels, again causing loss of energy and fatigue.

Inadequate dietary fiber has been associated with constipation, heart disease, diabetes, colon cancer, varicose veins, phlebitis and obesity.

A fat-deficient diet can result in eczema, achy joints, and

disorders of the skin and hair. A lack of essential fatty acids can affect concentration and memory, as well as mental energy.

Vitamin and mineral shortages can impair growth and maintenance of overall health, as well as mental and physical well-being.[16]

These same problems are thought to occur when we fail to digest our foods completely. Without complete digestion, many nutrients in our foods never make it to their intended destination—our body cells—and life becomes a slow hunger game. A person may be obese and still be deprived of certain nutritional elements.

And that's where the trouble starts.

What it all comes down to is this: Good nutrition is the key to maintaining homeostasis, where all cells are fully nourished, working in harmony, each doing its job, and contributing to the overall well-being of the organism, be it an amoeba, a household plant, or one of us.

It's the working enzymes that provide the fuel for our body cells by breaking down the foods we eat to useable, absorbable forms. Starch is useless until amylase breaks it down to glucose, at which point it enters the bloodstream and is used by the body cells as fuel. Again, the old saying that we are what we eat is not entirely true. We are what

we digest! All foods have to be broken down to their simplest components before the body cells can use them.

Gluten is a perfect example. Gluten is a protein that is rich in the amino acids proline and glutamine. These two amino acids bind together and can make gluten resistant to digestion and very inflammatory. But if you break the bond between these two amino acids and release glutamine, good things can happen. While hard-to-digest gluten causes spaces between the molecules in the intestinal lining to widen, resulting in leaky gut syndrome, glutamine tightens up these junctions so partially digested foods and bacterial toxins no longer leak into the bloodstream and cause body-wide inflammation.

Glutamine also happens to be one of the preferred fuels for the immune system's white blood cells.

So breaking up gluten and releasing glutamine helps keep our intestinal lining healthy, and it fuels our immune system. This is where protease supplements come in. In fact, one of the main enzymes currently being investigated for gluten intolerance is a plant-derived protease enzyme, from barley.

Again, it all comes down to complete digestion providing nourishment and fuel for the body cells to work in homeostatic harmony.

Again, if you don't digest your food, it's not available and not absorbed. It's that simple.

Proteins, carbohydrates, fats, vitamins, minerals, that double cheeseburger, it all has to be broken down to its most basic elements before any of it can be used by body cells for growth, repairs, and energy for body activities.

It seems obvious to say that if you are eating healthy and getting all the nutrients that your body cells need, your health should be maintained at a much higher level.

WHY FOOD ENZYME SUPPLEMENTS?

So why should we take food enzyme supplements? If nothing else, they're an insurance policy.

Because between cooking and processing, and the continuing quest for increased shelf life, there simply doesn't appear to be enough enzyme potential left in the foods we eat to do all the predigestive work that Nature intended.

Finally, recent science has shown that protease supplements actually perform systemic duties as well. After doing their digestive work, these hard-working enzymes are absorbed from the intestines and transported around the body by white blood cells and released to do their

work in areas of inflammation, where they may be needed.[17] So, in the end, supplemental enzymes appear to work in a number of ways to support and maintain our health.

They work in the food enzyme stomach to predigest the foods we eat, after which some of these supplemental troops continue working alongside the pancreatic enzymes in the small intestine. All of this is believed to take a lot of the burden off our overworked pancreas, and, as Howell believed, it may also help preserve our "enzyme potential" as we age.

Good predigestion means there's less need for the body to recruit white blood cells to assist in digestion and clean up the toxic mess resulting from bacterial overgrowth. Without a steady stream of toxins and partially digested food antigens making their way across our intestinal walls, the resulting inflammatory cascade becomes less of an issue. With less toxic rain falling on cell surfaces, inside blood vessels, joints, in every corporeal nook and cranny, without that bit of undigested burnt red meat finding its way into Dr. Coffey's little garden of good and evil, it would be logical to assume that there would be less risk for the degenerative diseases that have come to be associated with this inflammatory cascade—i.e., arthritis, heart disease and cancer.

WHAT SCIENCE IS REVEALING TODAY

It's all about inflammation.

Whenever we eat enzyme-deficient foods, we may be creating inflammation.

But if we eat less cooked and processed foods, and more fresh produce, and take enzyme supplements to achieve more complete digestion, this inflammatory cascade may be greatly reduced.

And our body cells should get more of the nutrients they need to work in homeostatic harmony.

Suddenly, the inflammatory cascade may be muted.

So let's ask the question again.

Can enzyme supplements, combined with good nutrition and portion control, and no smoking, help us live longer, healthier lives?

It appears this may be the case.

Maybe what this all comes down to is that food enzymes represent an insurance policy for maintaining optimal health. In the case of vitamin C, 100% of the daily value set forth by the FDA is 60 milligrams. That's to prevent vitamin C deficiency-related diseases, such as scurvy. On the other hand, it's been noted, the optimum value of vitamin C is at least 200 milligrams

per day, or possibly much higher to "maximize the vitamin's potential health benefits."[17] I don't know too many Americans who just want "average" health, but there are many Americans who would hope to "optimize" their health.

Enzyme supplements offer us the opportunity to achieve and maintain optimal health, even as Nature's enzymes continue to disappear from the foods we eat.

Doc Howell saw this years ago.

And once again, the science is suggesting he was right.

GLOSSARY

OF DIGESTIVE ENZYMES

A

ACTIVITY UNITS like IU for vitamin E, enzymes need to be labeled on the basis of their activity; each enzyme has a unique activity unit that measures its ability to break down a certain substance

AGU AmyloGlucosidase Units—FCC activity unit used to declare Glucoamylase activity

- **GALACTOSIDASE** enzyme that breaks down complex sugars found in beans, broccoli, cabbage and other vegetables that commonly cause bloating, gas, and flatulence; helps prevent gas

ALU Acid Lactase Units—FCC activity units used to declare Lactase activity

AP AminoPeptidase—FCC activity unit sometimes used to declare various protease activity

AMINO ACIDS the building blocks of proteins

AMYLASE enzymes that break down starch; when used for dietary supplements commonly refers to •-amylase activity

ANTIOXIDANT a compound that neutralizes oxidative substances

ASPERGILLUS common fungal microorganisms used to produce enzymes via fermentation

B

BACILLUS a bacteria that is commonly used to produce enzymes via fermentation

BAU Bacterial Amylase Unit—FCC activity unit used to declare bacterial a-Amylase activity

•-GLUCANASE enzyme that disrupts NSPs

BGU Beta-Glucanase Unit—FCC activity units used to declare •-Glucanase activity

BROMELAIN a protease from Pineapple (Ananas comosus) latex

C

CARBOHYDRASE any enzymes that break down sugar-based compounds known as carbohydrates

CARBOHYDRATES compounds made up of various sugars including simple sugars, disaccharides, trisaccharides and complex polysaccharides

CATALASE an antioxidant enzyme

CATALYST any substance capable of increasing the speed of chemical reactions

CELLULASE enzyme that breaks down cellulose

CELLULOSE common form of non-soluble fiber, these chains of glucose are not digested by human beings

CERECALASE. Our proprietary enzyme blend of three enzymes: Hemicellulase, beta-Glucanase and Phytase that break down various NSPs to help improve mineral release

CHYMOTRYPSIN a pancreatic protease that functions in the small intestine to digest proteins

CU Cellulase Units—FCC activity units used to declare cellulase activity

D

DIASTASE a mixture of amylases that includes both •-amylase and •-amylase; use in dietary supplements commonly signifies the presence of •-amylase activity

DIGESTION process by which food is broken down and absorbed; begins in the mouth and continues throughout the digestive tract

DISACCHARIDE a sugar made up of two simple sugars such as sucrose and lactose

DPo Degrees Diastatic Power—FCC activity unit for the declaration of total amylase activity of barley malt, diastase and other enzyme preparations

DU Dextrinizing Units—FCC activity units used to declare fungal •-amylase activity

E

ENZYME proteins that catalyze the biochemical reactions necessary for all life

EX VIVO a type of in vitro experiment conducted on intact tissues that have been removed from organisms such as muscle fibers

F

FATTY ACIDS when freed from their backbone, fatty acids are an important source of structural components and energy the body

FATS also called lipids, they are composed of a glycerol backbone and three fatty acids making a E-shaped compound; our bodies use fats for energy and to produce important biochemicals

FCC Food Chemical Codex—compendial text of testing methods for food chemicals; the current standard of activity for enzyme supplement labels

FIP—FCC activity units used to declare Lipase activity; this assay was adopted from the Federation Internationale Pharmaceutique compendium and bears its name

FTU FyTase Unit—FCC activity units used to declare Phytase activity

FUNGUS this large group of organisms includes yeasts, molds and mushrooms; many supplemental enzymes are produced by fermentation by different fungi

G

GALU •-Galactosidase Unit—FCC activity unit used to declare •-Galactisdase activity

GDU Gelatin Digesting Unit—activity unit sometimes used to declare protease activity including Bromelain

GERD Gastro Esophageal Reflux Disease

GASTRIC/GASTRO technical terms that refer to the stomach

GLUCOAMYLASE also known as amyloglucosidase, this enzyme works with amylase to break down starches

GLUCOSE a common simple sugar and the primary energy source of human cells

GLUTEN found in grains including wheat, barley and rye, these proteins are resistant to digestion by human proteases and can cause digestive discomfort, intolerance, allergy or Celiac Disease in some individuals

GLYCEROL the structural backbone of fats

GRAS FDA designation that a substance is Generally Regarded As Safe

H

HEMICELLULASE a group of enzymes that disrupts NSPs

HCL hydrochloric acid, produced by our stomachs to aid in the chemical digestion of food, it also activates the stomach protease known as pepsin

HCU HemiCellulase Unit—FCC activity unit used to declare Hemicellulase activity

HUT Hemoglobin Units on a Tyrosine basis—FCC activity units used to declare fungal Protease activity

HYDROLYSIS technical term that refers to the enzymatic digestion or break down of a substrate

I

IN VITRO experiment performed outside of a living organism to simulate conditions in the body under more controlled conditions

IN VIVO experiment carried out in a living organism; animal testing and clinical trials are two examples of in vivo studies

INVU INVertase Unit—activity unit used to declare Invertase (Sucrase) activity

ISOLASE. Our proprietary enzyme blend that removes the sugar from isoflavones to support improved availability of these bioactive compounds from soy and other botanicals

ISOU Isolase Unit—activity units used to declare the activity of the proprietary enzyme blend Isolase.

L

LACTASE enzyme that breaks down milk sugar into simple sugars

LACTOFERRIN amazing immune supporting protein with antioxidant, antimicrobial and proteolytic activity

LACTOPEROXIDASE an antioxidant enzyme first isolated from milk

LACTOSE milk sugar, a disaccharide made up of the simple sugars glucose and galactose

LIPASE enzyme that breaks down fats

LYSOZYME an antioxidant enzyme that also has potent antimicrobial action

M

MALTASE enzyme that breaks down the disaccharide maltose to produce two free glucose molecules

MU Macerating Units—activity units used to declare CereCalase activity

MCU Milk Clotting Unit—FCC activity unit sometimes used to declare activity of certain proteases including Papain

N

NATTOKINASE protease enzyme first isolated in the traditional fermented bean dish known as Natto; the enzyme functions systemically as a fibrinolytic to support cardiovascular health

NATTOZIMES. Our proprietary blend of proteases that has fibrinolytic activity similar to nattokinase

NSPS Non-Starch Polysaccharides—compounds other than starch made up of chains of simple sugars

P

PANCREATIN mammalian enzyme preparation produced by the pancreas that provides protease, lipase and amylase activity; requires enteric coating for survival through the stomach

PANCRELIPASE enzymes from mammalian pancreas that has a higher lipase content than pancreatin; requires enteric coating for survival through the stomach

PAPAIN a protease from papaya (Carica papaya) latex

PC Bacterial Protease Unit—FCC activity unit used to declare proteolytic activity from bacterial sources

PECTINASE a group of enzymes that breaks down NSPs known as pectins

PEPSIN protease produced by the stomach to begin protein digestion; requires an acid environment for activation

PEPTIDASE enzyme that breaks down proteins into smaller pieces and free amino acids; while synonymous with "Protease" it is typically used in the supplement industry to identify an enzyme capable of increasing the release of free amino acids

PHYTASE enzyme that breaks down phytic acid releasing phosphorus and bound minerals

PHYTONUTRIENTS generic term for compounds from plants that have beneficial effects on the human body

POLYSACCHARIDE a complex carbohydrate made up of chains of sugars; example include starch and cellulose

PROBIOTIC living microorganisms, which when consumed, colonize our intestines and provide many benefits, supporting digestion and our immune systems

PROTEASE enzyme that breaks down proteins into smaller pieces and free amino acids

PROTEIN chains of amino acids, our bodies use proteins for many different things from communication to building muscle and even making more enzymes

PU Papain Unit—FCC activity units commonly used to declare proteolytic activity from plant proteases

R

RHIZOPUS fungal microorganisms used to produce enzymes via fermentation

S

SACCHAROMYCES yeast used to produce enzymes, primarily invertase, via fermentation

SAP Spectrophotometric Acid Protease—FCC activity units used to declare fungal protease activity

SERRAPEPTIDASE enzyme originally isolated from a bacteria, Serratia marcescens, in the gut of silk worms; protease with systemic applications supporting immune and cardiovascular health; synonymous with serratiopeptidase and serrapeptase

SERRAZIMES. NEC's proprietary blend of proteases that has activity similar to serrapeptidase

STARCH simple chains of glucose, easily digested by most human beings

SU Sumner Unit—FCC activity unit used to declare Invertase (Sucrase) activity

SUBSTRATE technical term for whatever compound with which a given enzyme reacts; for example, protein is the substrate of protease

SUCROSE table sugar, a disaccharide made up of the simple sugars glucose and fructose

SOD Super Oxide Dismutase—an antioxidant enzyme

SYSTEMIC ENZYMES taken on an empty stomach for nutritional benefits beyond the digestive tract often composed of proteolytic enzymes

T

TRICHODERMA fungal microorganisms used to produce enzymes via fermentation

TRYPSIN a pancreatic protease that functions in the small intestine to digest proteins

U

USP United States Pharmacopeia—compendial text for pharmaceutical testing methods; also activity unit for most animal-derived digestive enzymes including Pancreatin, Pancrelipase, Pepsin, Trypsin, and Chymotrypsin

X

XYLANASE an enzyme that breaks down NSPs known as xylans

List provided by the National Enzyme Company website at http://www.nationalenzyme.com

REFERENCES

BY CHAPTER

CHAPTER I

[1] Bear, Marjorie Warvelle (2007). *A Square Mile of Chicago* (Oak Brook, IL: TIPRAC), p. 266.

[2] Elmhurst Historical Museum. *The Lindlahr Sanitarium.* Retrieved from http://www.elmhurst.org/DocumentCenter/Home/View/261.

[3] Fishman, Stanley A. (2011). *More Blessings From Pastured Butter.* Retrieved from http://www.tendergrassfedmeat.com/tag/butter-for-healing/.

[4] Bennett, Joan W. (2001). Adrenalin and cherry trees. *Modern Drug Discovery,* vol. 4, no. 12, pp 47-48, 51. Retrieved from http://pubs.acs.org/subscribe/archive/mdd/v04/i12/html/12timeline.html.

[5] Bear, 2007, *op. cit.,* p. 267.

CHAPTER 2

[1] National Library of Medicine, National Institutes of Health (2014). Enzyme definition. Retrieved from http://ghr.nlm.nih.gov/glossary=enzyme.

[2] Howell, Edward (1985). *Enzyme Nutrition: The Food Enzyme Concept* (Garden City, NY: Avery Publishing Group), p. 1.

[3] Howell, 1985, *ibid.,* p. 33.

[4] Howell, Edward (1994). *Food Enzymes for Health and Longevity* (Twin Lakes, WI: Lotus Press), p. 215.

[5] Lopez, D.A., Williams, R.M., & Miehlke, M. (1994). *Enzymes: The Fountain of Life* (Newark, DE: Neville Press), p. 63.

[6] Lopez et al., 1994, *ibid.,* p. 69.

[7] Loomis, Howard F., Jr., 1999. *Enzymes: The Key to Health* (Madison, WI: 21st Century Nutrition Publishing), p. 74.

[8] Lopez et al., 1994, *op. cit.,* p 6.

[9] Lopez et al., 1994, *op. cit.,* p. 57.

[10] Retrieved from http://www.novozymes.com/en/about-us/our-business/what-are-enzymes/Pages/finding-and-producing-enzymes.aspx.

CHAPTER 3

[1] Howell, Edward (1994). *Food Enzymes for Health and Longevity* (Twin Lakes, WI: Lotus Press).

[2] Howell, Edward (1985). *Enzyme Nutrition: The Food Enzyme Concept* (Garden City, NJ: Avery Publishing Group), p. 4.

[3] Howell, 1985, *ibid.,* p. 2.

[4] Howell, 1985, *ibid.,* p. 13.

[5] Howell, 1985, *ibid.,* p. 13.

[6] Howell, 1985, *ibid.,* p. 8.

[7] Howell, 1985, *ibid.,* pp. 148, 161.

[8] Howell, 1985, *ibid.,* p. 150.

[9] Thomas, William A. (1927). Health of a carnivorous race: a study of the Eskimo. *Journal of the American Medical Association,* vol. 88, no. 20, pp. 1559-1560.

[10] Howell, 1985, *op. cit.,* pp. 46, 150, 152.

[11] *Biochemistry,* vol. xxxi, 1937, p. 343) (*Time Magazine,* May 18, 1936)

[12] Howell, 1985, *op. cit.,* p. 153.

[13] Howell, 1985, *op. cit.,* p. 47.

[14] Elvevoll, E.O., & Ostend, B. (2003). Impact of processing on nutritional quality of marine food items. *Forum of Nutrition*, vol. 56, pp. 337-340.

[15] Howell, 1985, *op. cit.,* p. 17.

[16] Howell, 1994, *op. cit.,* p. 25.

[17] Howell, 1985, *op. cit.,* p. 10.

[18] Beazell, James M., Ivy, A.C., & Schmidt, C.R. (1936). On the effectiveness of malt amylase on the astric digestion of starches. *Journal of Nutrition*, vol. 12, no, 1, pp. 59-83.

[19] Howell, 1985, *op. cit.*, p. 64.

[20] Howell, 1985, *op. cit.*, p. 5.

[21] Walkowiak, et al. (2011). The elimination of meat from the diet selectively decreases pancreatic elastase secretion. *British Journal of Nutrition,* vol. 98, pp. 154-158.

[22] Howell, 1985, *op. cit.*, p. 66.

[23] Perlmutter, David, Loberg, K. (2013). *Grain Brain* (New York, NY: Little, Brown and Company), pp. 182-184.

[24] Howell, 1985, *op. cit.*, p. 73.

[25] Howell, 1985, *op. cit.*, p. 7.

[26] Howell, 1985, *op. cit.*, p. xi.

[27] Howell, 1985, *op. cit.*, p. 73.

[28] Howell, 1985, op. cit., p. 40.

[29] Retrieved from http://deltatrak.com/index.php/produce-shelf-life-issues-and-extension-methods-from-harvest-to-retailer.

[30] Retrieved from http://www.arcadiabio.com/extendedshelflife.

CHAPTER 4

[1] Coffey, Don, & De Marzo, Angelo (2000). Evolution and prostate cancer. *Prostate Cancer Discovery*, vol. V. Retrieved from http://urology.jhu.edu/newsletter/prostate_cancer511.php.

[2] Coffey, D.S. (2001). Similarities of prostate and breast cancer: evolution, diet and estrogens. *Urology,* vol. 57, no. 4A, pp. 31-38.

[3] Pottenger, Francis Marion, Jr. (1995). *Pottenger's Cats: A Study in Nutrition* (Lemon Grove, CA: Price-Pottenger Nutrition Foundation).

[4] Little, Susan (2005). Managing chronic diseases in cats. Retrieved from DVM360.com.

[5] Howell, Edward (1994). *Food Enzymes for Health and Longevity* (Twin Lakes, WI: Lotus Press), p. 120.

[6] Fox, Herbert (1923). *Disease in Captive Wild Mammals and Birds: Incidence, Description, Comparison* (Philadelphia, PA: J.B. Lippincott Company).

[7] Fox, 1923, *ibid.*, p. 179.

[8] Howell, 1994, *op. cit.*, p. 120.

[9] Howell, 1994, *op. cit.*, p. 123.

[10] *Vet J*, vol. 90, 1934, pp. 368-374.

[11] Howell, 1994, *op. cit.*, p. 148.

[12] Howell, Edward (1985). *Enzyme Nutrition: The Food Enzyme Concept* (Garden City, NJ: Avery Publishing Group), p. 6.

[13] Howell, 1994, *op. cit.*, p. 55.

[14] Howell, 1985, *op. cit.*, p. 84.

[15] Loomis, 1999, *op. cit.*, p. 68.

[16] Blake, William. *Auguries of Innocence.* Retrieved from http://www.poetryfoundation.org/poem/172906.

[17] Loomis, 1999, *op. cit.*, pp. 108, 102.

[18] Loomis, 1999, *op. cit.*, p. 110.

[19] Loomis, 1999, *op. cit.*, p. 104.

CHAPTER 5

[1] U.S. Department of Health and Human Services (1988). *The Surgeon General's Report on Nutrition and Health* (Washington, DC: U.S. Department of Health and Human Services, Public Health Service), HHS (PHS) Publication No. 88-50210.

[2] Loomis, Howard F., Jr. (1999). *Enzymes: The Key to Health* (Madison, WI: 21st Century Nutrition Publishing), p. 111.

[3] Loomis, 1999, *ibid.*, p. 112.

[4] Rogers, Kara, ed. (2011). *Blood Physiology and Circulation* (Chicago, IL: Britannica Educational Publishing), p. 198.

[5] Kouchakoff, P. (1930). The influence of food cooking on the blood formula of man. *Proceedings: First International Congress of Microbiology,* Paris, 1930. Translation by Lee Foundation for Nutritional Research. Milwaukee, WI.

[6] Paganelli, R., Matricardi, P.M., Aiuti, F. (1984) Interactions of food antigens, antibodies, and antigen-antibody complexes in health and disease. *Clinical Reviews in Allergy,* February 1984, Vol. 2, Issue 1, pp. 69-78.

[7] Heyman M., Desjeux, J.F. (December 2000). Cytokine-Induced Alteration of the Epithelial Barrier to Food Antigens in Disease. *Annals of the New York Academy of Sciences,* Vol. 915, pp. 304-311.

[8] Kouchakoff, P. (1937). Nouvelles lois de l'alimentation humaine basées sur la leucocytose digestive (F. Rouge & Cie SA).

[9] Husby, S. (1988). Dietary antigens: uptake and humoral immunity in man. *APMIS Supplement*, vol. 1, pp. 1-40.

[10] 8) *Science Magazine* (2013), Special Issue on Inflammation, vol. 339, no. 6116; *Nature,* article on inflammation, vol. 454, no. 7203, pp. 427-477.

[11] Loomis, 1999, *op. cit.,* p. 74.

[12] Lopez, D.A., Williams, R.M., & Miehlke, M. (1994). *Enzymes: The Fountain of Life* (Newark, DE: Neville Press), p. 150.

[13] Loomis, Howard F., Jr. (1999). *Enzymes: The Key to Health,* (Madison, WI: 21st Century Nutrition Publishing), p. 122.

[14] Zhao, Xiaoyan, et al. Circulating immune complexes contain citrullinated fibrinogen in rheumatoid arthritis. *Arthritis Research & Therapy*, vol. 10, no. 4.

[15] Levinsky, R.J. (1978). Role of circulating soluble immune complexes in disease. *Archives of Disease in Childhood*, pp. 96–99)

[16] McMahon, Maureen, et al. (2007). Atherosclerosis and systemic lupus erythematosus—mechanistic basis of the association. *Current Opinions in Immunology*, vol. 19, no. 6, pp. 633-639.

[17] Mustafa, Awder, et al. (2000). Circulating immune complexes in 50-year-old men as a strong and independent risk factor for myocardial infarction. *Circulation*, vol. 102, pp. 2576-2581.

[18] Erridge, C. (2010). The capacity of foodstuffs to induce innate immune activation of human monocytes *in vitro* is dependent on food content of stimulants of Toll-like receptors 2 and 4. *British Journal of Nutrition*, vol. 20; pp. 1-9.

[19] Stokowski, L.A. (June 20, 2013). Red meat and cancer: What's the beef? Medscape, June 20, 2013. Retrieved from http://www.medscape.com/viewarticle/806573.

[20] Joshi, A.D., Corral, R., Catsburg, C., et al. (2012). Red meat and poultry, cooking practices, genetic susceptibility, and risk of prostate cancer: results from a multiethnic case-control study. Carcinogenesis, vol. 33, pp. 2108-2118.

[21] Corpet, D. (2011). Red meat and colon cancer: Should we become vegetarians, or can we make meat safer? *Meat Science,* vol. 89, pp. 310-316.

[22] Chan, D.S., Lau, R., Aune, D., et al. (2011). Red and processed meat and colorectal cancer incidence: meta-analysis of prospective studies. *PLoS One,* vol. 6, p. e20456

[23] Wu, J.W., Cross, A.J., Baris, D., et al. (2012). Dietary intake of meats, fruits, vegetables, and selective micronutrients and risk of bladder cancer in the New England region of the United States. *British Journal of Cancer,* vol. 106, pp. 1891-1898.

[24] Daniel, C.R., Cross, A.J., Graubard, B.L., et al. (2012). Large prospective investigation of meat intake, related mutagens, and risk of renal cell carcinoma. *American Journal of Clinical Nutrition,* vol. 95, pp. 155-162.

[25] Yang, W.S., Wong, M.Y., Vogtmann, E., et al. Meat consumption and risk of lung cancer: evidence from observational studies. *Annals of Oncology,* vol. 23, pp. 3163-3170.

[26] Rohrmann, S., Overvad, K., Bueno-de-Mesquita, H.B., et al. (2013). Meat consumption and mortality—results from the European Prospective Investigation into Cancer and Nutrition. *BMC Medicine,* vol. 11, p. 63.

[27] Pan, A., Sun, Q., Bernstein, A.M., et al. (2012). Red meat consumption and mortality: results from two prospective cohort studies. *Archives of Internal Medicine,* vol. 172, no. 7, pp. 555-563.

CHAPTER 6

[1] Howell, Edward (1985). *Enzyme Nutrition: The Food Enzyme Concept* (Garden City, NJ: Avery Publishing Group), p. 27.

[2] Howell, 1985, *ibid.,* p. 27.

[3] Leaf, Alexander (1973). Search for the oldest people. *National Geographic,* vol. 143, no. 1, pp. 93-118.

4 Moss, Ralph (2008). Enzymes, trophoblasts, and cancer: the afterlife of an idea (1924-2008). *Integrative Cancer Therapies,* vol. 7, pp. 262-275.

[5] Lopez, D.A., Williams, R.M., & Miehlke, M. (1994). *Enzymes: The Fountain of Life* (Newark, DE: Neville Press), p. 230.

[6] Leipner, Jorg, & Saller, Reinhard. (2000). Systemic enzyme therapy in oncology: effect and mode of action. *Drugs,* vol. 59, no. 4, pp. 769-780.

[7] Lopez et al., 1994, *op. cit.,* p. 135.

[8] Lopez et al., 1994, *op. cit.,* p. 233.

[9] Retrieved from http://www.ncbi.nlm.nih.gov/pubmed/10783488#.

[10] Dresser, L., & Rehberger, A. (1990). Induction of tumor necrosis factor in human peripheral-blood mononuclear cells by proteolytic enzymes. Oncology, vol. 47, pp. 475-477.

[11] Lopez et al., 1994, *op. cit.,* p. 235.

[12] Moss, 2008, *op. cit.*

[13] Lopez et al., 1994, *op. cit.,* p. 242.

[14] Lopez et al., 1994, *op. cit.,* p. 20.

[15] Adams, C.W.M., et al. (1962). A hypothesis to explain the accumulation of cholesterol in atherosclerosis. *The Lancet,* vol. 279, no. 7235, pp. 890-892.

[16] Rubenstein, Lucien J., et al. (1968). Experimental cerebral atherosclerosis in dogs. *Annals of the New York Academy of Sciences,* vol. 149, pp.

[17] Lopez et al., 1994, *op. cit.*, p. 222.

[18] Kasim, M., et al., (2009). Improved myocardial perfusion in stable angina pectoris by oral lumbrokinase: a pilot study. *Journal of Alternative and Complementary Medicine*, vol. 15, no. 5, pp. 539-544.

[19] Renshaw, Arnold (1947). Intestinal extract in rheumatic diseases. *Annals of the Rheumatic Diseases*, vol. 6, pp. 15-35.

[20] Howell, Edward (1994). *Food Enzymes for Health and Longevity* (Twin Lakes, WI: Lotus Press), p. 11.

[21] Lopez et al., 1994, *op. cit.*, p. 179.

[22] Akhtar, N.M., et al. (2004). Oral enzyme combination versus diclofenac in the treatment of osteoarthritis of the knee—a double-blind prospective randomized study. *Clinical Rheumatology*, vol. 23, no. 5.

[23] Zuschlag, J.M. (1988). Double-blind clinical study using certain proteolytic enzyme mixtures in karate fighters. Working paper. *Mucos Pharma GmbH (Germany)*, pp. 1-5.

[24] Baumuller, M. (1990). The application of hydrolytic enzymes in blunt wounds to the soft tissue and distortion of the ankle joint: a double-blind clinical trial [translated from German]. *Allgemeinmedizin*, vol. 19, pp. 178-182.

[25] Lopez et al., 1994, *op. cit.*, p. 203.

[26] Lopez et al., 1994, *op. cit.*, p. 206.

[27] Brudnak, Mark A., Rimland, B., Kerry, R.E. (2003). Beneficial effects of enzyme-based therapy for autism spectrum disorders. *Townsend Letter for Doctors & Patients*, October 2003.

[28] Retrieved from http://www.clinicaltrials.gov/ct2/show/NCT00881452?term=Curemark&rank=1.

[29] Retrieved from http://www.prnewswire.com/news-releases/curemark-to-enroll-children-9-12-years-of-age-into-medical-trial-of-cm-at-for-children-with-autism-165128016.html.

[30] Howell, 1985, op. cit., p. 65.

[31] Lopez et al., 1994, op. cit., p. 43.

CHAPTER 7

[1] Loomis, Howard F., Jr. (1999). *Enzymes: The Key to Health* (Madison, WI: 21st Century Nutrition Publishing), p. 79.

[2] Howell, Edward (1985). *Enzyme Nutrition: The Food Enzyme Concept* (Garden City, NJ: Avery Publishing Group), p. 115.

[3] Retrieved from http://www.webmd.com/diet/features/the-truth-about-starch-blockers.

[4] Kessler, Brad. (2009). *Goat Song: A Seasonal Life, a Short History of Herding, and the Art of Making Cheese* (New York, NY: Scribner), p. 163.

[5] Howell, 1985, *op. cit.,* p. 99.

[6] Retrieved from http://www.raw-milk-facts.com/raw_milk_health_benefits.html.

[7] Dahmani-Mardas F., Troadec, C., Boualem, A., et al. (2010). A: Engineering melon plants with improved fruit shelf life using the TILLING approach. *PloS ONE,* 5(12):e15776.

[8] Hendren, Reba K., *Canning Foods: Fruits, Vegetables, Pickles, Jellies* (Knoxville, TN: University of Tennessee, Institute of Agriculture), p. 3. Retrieved from https://ag.tennessee.edu/foodscience/Documents/Canning%20foods.pdf.

[9] Retrieved from http://www.gastro.org.

[10] Guarner, F., et al. (2008). *Map of Digestive Disorders and Diseases* (Milwaukee, WI: World Gastroenterology Organization).

[11] Retrieved from http://www.drugs.com/news/abbvie-survey-majority-americans-living-gi-48744.html.

[12] Loomis, 1999, *op. cit.,* p. 68.

[13] Howell, 1985, *op. cit.,* p. 11.

[14] Onetti, V., et al. (2010). The effect of oral supplementation with Lactobacillus reuteri or tilactase in lactose intolerant patients: randomized trial. *European Review for Medical and Pharmacological Sciences,* vol. 14, no. 3, pp. 163-170.

[15] Stepniak, D. (2006). Highly efficient gluten degradation with a newly identified prolyl endoprotease: implications for celiac disease. *American Journal of Physiology - Gastrointestinal and Liver Physiology,* vol. 291, no. 4, pp. G621-629.

[16] Loomis, 1999, *op. cit.,* p. 59.

[17] Lorkowski, Gerhard (2012). Gastrointestinal absorption and biological activities of serine and cysteine proteases of animal and plant origin: review on absorption of serine and cysteine proteases. *International Journal of Physiology, Pathophysiology and Pharmacology,* vol. 4, no. 1, pp. 10-27.

[18] Frei, B., et al., (2012). Authors' perspective: What is the optimum intake of vitamin C in humans? *Critical Reviews in Food Science and Nutrition*, vol. 52, no. 9, pp. 815-829.

INDEX

A

B

C

D

E

F

G

H

I

J

K

L

M

N

O

P

R

u

v

W

Y

Z

ACKNOWLEDGMENTS

The authors wish to express a special thanks to Anthony Collier, CEO of the National Enzyme Company, whose personal recollections have helped bring Dr. Edward Howell and his work to life in these pages. Additional thanks go to Dr. Howard Loomis for his help in bringing the science in these pages into such sharp focus. Finally, we wish to thank Meredith Pond, Jessica Koman, and Suzie Sutherland for their ongoing efforts in bringing this project to completion.

ABOUT THE AUTHORS

Paul M. Nemiroff, PhD, MD, FACS

Dr. Paul Nemiroff is a nationally recognized surgeon who received his MD degree from UCLA, with surgical residencies at UCLA/Cedars-Sinai and the University of Florida. He also holds a PhD from Purdue University in Administrative and Behavioral Sciences. Over the years, he has published and presented hundreds of articles and research papers on surgical techniques, the psychology of decision making, the healing benefits of hyperbaric oxygen, and also complementary medical therapies. He has performed over 10,000 surgeries.

An award-winning TV medical correspondent, Dr. Nemiroff is also the recipient of more than a dozen awards, including one from the American Cancer Society. He was invited to Washington, DC, where he was considered a candidate for Surgeon General of the United States.

Arnold Mann

Arnold Mann has been writing about medicine for 30 years. His cover stories for *TIME* and *USA Weekend Magazine* have earned him recognition as one of the nation's leading medical journalists. Mr. Mann served as co-author of Dr. Keith Black's book, *Brain Surgeon: A Doctor's Inspiring Encounters with Mortality and Miracles* (Grand Central Publishing, 2010), which was nominated for an NAACP Image Award (Best Nonfiction Book).

Mr. Mann has also written extensively for publications of the National Institutes of Health. He served as personal writer for the Director of the National Cancer Institute, and he oversaw publication of the Institute's *Annual Progress Report to Congress.*

Made in the USA
Monee, IL
27 March 2026

47094580R00138